Pathology:
Review for New National Boards

Pathology:
Review for New National Boards

Frank N. Miller, M. D.
Professor Emeritus of Pathology
The George Washington University Medical Center
Washington, D.C.

J&S

J&S Publishing Company Inc., Alexandria, Virginia

J&S

Composition and Layout: Ronald C. Bohn, Ph. D.
Cover Design: Kurt E. Johnson, Ph. D.
Printing Supervisor: Robert Perotti, Jr.
Printing: Goodway Graphics, Springfield, Virginia

Library of Congress Catalog Card Number 93-079828

ISBN 0-9632873-3-8

Dedication

Frank N. Miller would like to dedicate this book to Caroline, Catherine, and Donald.

Table of Contents

Preface . . . . *vii*

Acknowledgements . . . . *viii*

Chapter I   *General Pathology* *1*

Chapter II   *Cardiovascular Pathology* *55*

Chapter III   *Hematological and Lymphatic Pathology, Immunopathology* *75*

Chapter IV   *Respiratory Pathology* *103*

Chapter V   *Digestive System Pathology* *119*

Chapter VI   *Urinary System Pathology* *139*

Chapter VII   *Reproductive System Pathology* *155*

Chapter VIII *Endocrine Pathology* *177*

Chapter IX   *Nervous System Pathology* *189*

Chapter X   *Musculoskeletal, Cutaneous, and Sensory Pathology* *203*

Preface

This book is designed to enable you to review in just 1-2 days all of the basic pathology you studied in the second year of medical school: General Pathology, Inflammation and Neoplasia, Infectious Disease, and Organ System Pathology. We have been able to condense a review of all basic pathology into a single book because of the new format of the National Board Part I Exam. It is no longer prudent to review exhaustively the basic science courses because the new examination format no longer rewards an encyclopedic knowledge of the basic sciences. Instead, the new exams test knowledge of the scientific basis of disease and the ability to apply basic scientific information to the clinical reasoning process. Consequently, the most efficient way to study for the new exam is 1) to review only the most clinically relevant material from each basic science course and 2) to focus on the application of this material to the solution of clinical problems. These two new study features form the core of this text.

If you answer every question and read all the tutorials in this book, you can cover within 1-2 days all of the most clinically relevant information from your basic pathology course. You will find that many pathologic facts reviewed or learned anew will be presented in the context of a clinical case or an illustration. We hope that the clinical cases and illustrations will enhance your understanding and recall of the information. Many tutorials begin with short, specific comments on the answers to the preceding Items. This material is contained in a lined box. It is followed by a more detailed but concise discussion of the pathologic concepts dealt with in the Items. Thus, the reader may use the questions as a quick review by referring only to the boxed material or as a more extensive review of Pathology by reading the basic information in the more comprehensive discussions. Finally, you will learn from the tutorials how pathologic information is used by knowledgeable physicians to understand the courses of diseases and the significance of abnormal findings.

Frank N. Miller
Washington, D.C.
August, 1993

Acknowledgements

The author would like to thank Kurt E. Johnson, Ph. D., Professor, Department of Anatomy, The George Washington University Medical Center for his invaluable editorial assistance and Ronald C. Bohn, Ph. D., Associate Professor, Department of Anatomy, The George Washington University Medical Center for his skillful manipulation of the final documents for publication. Louis DePalma, M.D., Associate Professor of Pathology and Anatomy, Chief, Hematopathology, The George Washington University Medical Center, graciously read the manuscript. The author is grateful for all of this help and acknowledges any errors in this book as his own.

Disclaimer

The clinical information presented in this book is accurate for the purposes of review for licensure examinations but in no way should be used to treat patients or substituted for modern clinical training. Proper diagnosis and treatment of patients requires comprehensive evaluation of all symptoms, careful monitoring for adverse responses to treatment and assessment of the long-term consequences of therapeutic intervention.

CHAPTER I

GENERAL PATHOLOGY

Items 1-6

A middle-aged homeless man was found unconscious on the street and died shortly after admission to the hospital. The cause of death was acute liver failure. A photomicrograph of the liver at autopsy is shown in Figure 1.1

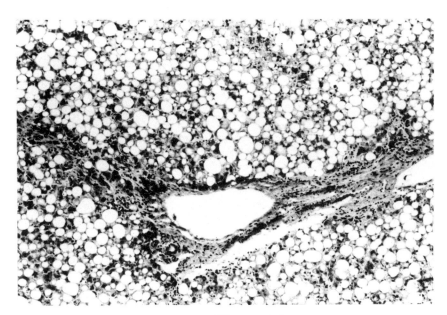

Figure 1.1

1.   The most likely pathologic process shown is

    (A)   cloudy swelling
    (B)   coagulation necrosis
    (C)   fatty degeneration
    (D)   hydropic degeneration
    (E)   inflammation

2. The lipid in hepatic cells in fatty degeneration is mainly in the form of

   (A) cholesterol esters
   (B) fatty acids
   (C) lipoproteins
   (D) phospholipids
   (E) triglycerides

3. The commonest cause of fatty change in the liver is

   (A) anemia
   (B) chloroform
   (C) ethyl alcohol
   (D) hypercholesterolemia
   (E) toxemia of pregnancy

4. If the patient had survived and continued to drink alcohol heavily, he would have been prone to develop

   (A) cirrhosis of the liver
   (B) hepatic abscess
   (C) hepatocarcinoma
   (D) nodular hyperplasia of the liver
   (E) viral hepatitis

5. Cloudy swelling is due to an increase in intracellular

   (A) calcium
   (B) endoplasmic reticulum
   (C) lipid
   (D) potassium
   (E) water

6. Hydropic degeneration of the renal tubular epithelium occurs in

   (A) chronic alcoholism
   (B) carbon tetrachloride poisoning
   (C) excessive renal sodium loss
   (D) hypokalemia
   (E) mercury poisoning

ANSWERS AND TUTORIAL ON ITEMS 1-6

The answers are: **1-C; 2-E; 3-C; 4-A; 5-E; 6-D**.

In Item 1, grossly, this liver was yellow and enlarged. The microscopic changes are characteristic of fatty degeneration. The lipid in hepatocytes in fatty change is mainly in the form of triglycerides. The commonest cause is ethyl alcohol poisoning. Continued excessive use of alcohol commonly leads to hepatic cirrhosis.

Cloudy swelling is due to failure of the cellular sodium pump. This allows excess sodium to enter cells and eventually increases cellular water. Hydropic degeneration is a severe form of cloudy swelling. It occurs with hypokalemia due to vomiting or diarrhea.

When the cells of an organ are affected diffusely by an adverse circumstance, as by bacterial toxins or inadequate oxygen supply, the affected organ is increased in size and weight. The tissues lose their normal glistening translucency and resemble boiled meat. This is cloudy swelling caused by an increase in intracellular water due to injury to the plasma membrane and mitochondria. The mitochondrial damage leads to decreased oxidative phosphorylation and ATP production. Sodium enters the cells in increased amounts and draws in water. Chiefly affected are certain highly specialized cells such as the epithelial cells of the convoluted tubules of the kidneys and hepatocytes. Affected cells are swollen, and fine granules and vacuoles can be seen in the cytoplasm. Nuclei are usually not affected.

Hydropic (vacuolar) degeneration results from a more severe degree of water imbibition into the cell cytoplasm. It occurs in some severe bacterial infections with high fever, certain types of poisoning, and hypokalemia. Potassium is drawn from cells and replaced by sodium and water in large amounts. In its most striking form, hydropic degeneration involves the renal tubular epithelium. Translucent intracytoplasmic vacuoles, which may be so large as to push the nucleus against the plasma membrane, appear in the proximal convoluted tubular cells. The vacuoles represent great accumulations of water in the endoplasmic reticulum, Golgi, and mitochondria.

Fatty degeneration (fatty metamorphosis, fatty change, steatosis) is the abnormal appearance of fat within parenchymal cells. Fat vacuoles may accumulate in liver cells under either physiologic or pathologic conditions. The physiologic type of fatty liver may occur after a fatty meal. The pathologic type of fatty liver may occur as a result of poisoning by hepatotoxic agents such as ethyl alcohol, chloroform, or carbon tetrachloride, during severe infections, in prolonged anemia, and in toxemia of pregnancy. The defect in the pathologic type of fatty liver may be a reduction in the capability of the liver cells to synthesize the phospholipid or protein moiety of lipoprotein; decreased lipoprotein release from hepatocytes; or increased triglyceride production. As a consequence, lipid accumulates in the liver cells, mainly in the form of triglycerides.

Items 7-10

A 60 year-old man developed urinary frequency and retention. Rectal examination revealed a firm, nodular, enlarged prostate. A photomicrograph of the surgically resected gland is shown in Figure 1.2.

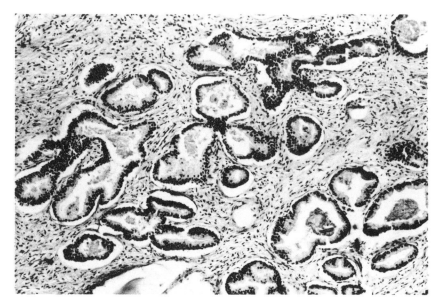

Figure 1.2

7. The pathologic process shown in this photomicrograph is

    (A) anaplasia
    (B) dysplasia
    (C) hyperplasia
    (D) hypertrophy
    (E) metaplasia

8. Urethral obstruction of long standing due to prostatic enlargement leads to which of the following changes in the urinary bladder muscularis?

    (A) atrophy
    (B) dysplasia
    (C) hyperplasia
    (D) hypertrophy
    (E) metaplasia

4

9. Urethral obstruction of long standing leads to which of the following pathological changes in the kidneys?

    (A)   atrophy
    (B)   dysplasia
    (C)   hyperplasia
    (D)   hypertrophy
    (E)   metaplasia

10. The replacement of cells by a type different from that normally found is

    (A)   anaplasia
    (B)   dysplasia
    (C)   hyperplasia
    (D)   metaplasia
    (E)   neoplasia

ANSWERS AND TUTORIAL ON ITEMS 7-10

The answers are: **7-C; 8-D; 9-A; 10-D**.

> In men over 50, the prostate gland frequently develops hyperplasia of the glandular epithelium and stroma, resulting in enlargement of the lateral and median lobes. In some cases urethral obstruction occurs, resulting in hypertrophy of the urinary bladder muscularis, with thickening and trabeculation of the vesical wall. Prolonged back-pressure from the urinary obstruction causes dilatation of the ureters and renal pelves and calyces. The renal parenchyma becomes atrophic as a result of the long term back-pressure.

Hyperplasia is an increase in the number of cells of a part. Hyperplasia may occur in response to chronic irritation or to endocrine stimulation, or it may be compensatory. It is present in certain viral diseases, such as molluscum contagiosum. It occurs in reverting postmitotic and intermitotic cells.

Hypertrophy is an increase in the size of individual cells or fibers so that an organ is enlarged. It occurs in postmitotic cells. There is no increase in the number of cells or fibers. True hypertrophy occurs in response to some demand for increased function. Physiologic hypertrophy develops apart from disease; e.g., the pregnant uterus and the muscles of athletes or laborers. Adaptive hypertrophy occurs in hollow viscera when the outlet is partly obstructed, the wall becoming thickened from enlargement of the muscle fibers; e.g., the left ventricle in aortic stenosis. In hypertrophic muscle cells, there is an increase in the number of myofilaments and mitochondria and the amount of endoplasmic reticulum.

Atrophy is an acquired decrease in size of a portion of the body, an organ, a tissue, or individual cells. The reduction in size in a part may be due to a decrease in the number of its structural units or in the size of the individual units, or both. The unspecialized connective tissues are less affected than parenchymal cells, so that the former often appear relatively increased. Besides, there is frequently fibrous or fatty replacement of lost elements.

Metaplasia occurs when a type of cell different from that normally found in a given location is produced. It is a reversible process. Epithelial metaplasia usually consists of the replacement of columnar epithelium by stratified squamous epithelium. It is commonly found in the bronchi of cigarette smokers. Connective tissue metaplasia occurs mainly in foci of chronic inflammation, especially where there has been necrosis and calcification.

Dysplasia is a change in mature cells in which their normal relationships to each other are disturbed and the cells show variations in size, shape, and nuclear characteristics. Some cases of dysplasia progress to malignant neoplasia. Common sites of dysplasia are the lip, the bronchi in cigarette smokers, and the cervix uteri.

Malignant neoplasms are characterized microscopically by a pronounced distortion of tissue pattern. The most conspicuous changes are variations in cell size and shape; increase in nuclear size, shape and staining qualities; and increase in frequency of mitotic figures, some or many of which may be tripolar or otherwise abnormal. These microscopic alterations collectively are known as anaplasia.

Items 11-15

In Items 11-14, match each disorder with the type of necrosis typically associated with it.

        (A)   caseation necrosis
        (B)   coagulation necrosis
        (C)   fat necrosis
        (D)   fibrinoid necrosis
        (E)   liquefaction necrosis

11.   obstruction of arterial blood supply

12.   leakage of pancreatic enzymes

13.   histoplasmosis

14.   infarct of cerebrum

15.   Metastatic calcification results from

        (A)   fat necrosis
        (B)   fracture of a bone
        (C)   hypercalcemia
        (D)   malignant neoplasia
        (E)   miliary tuberculosis

ANSWERS AND TUTORIAL ON ITEMS 11-15

The answers are: **11-B; 12-C; 13-A; 14-E; 15-C**.

In most organs, obstruction of the blood supply leads to coagulation necrosis due to anoxia. In acute pancreatitis, leakage of lipase causes fat necrosis within adipose tissue. As in tuberculosis, a cell mediated immune reaction may cause caseation necrosis in histoplasmosis. Unlike infarcts in other organs which show coagulation necrosis, brain and spinal cord infarcts are characterized by liquefaction necrosis. Fibrinoid necrosis is due to localization of soluble immune complexes on arterial walls. Metastatic calcification occurs in normal tissues due to hypercalcemia, as opposed to dystrophic calcification in which calcium salts are deposited in previously damaged tissues.

Cellular degeneration becomes cellular necrosis when the point of irreversibility is reached in the degenerative process. Cell necrosis results from the death of a group of cells as a result of injurious influences, while the cells are still on contact with the living body. Any harmful influence capable of causing injury to cells may cause necrosis. Usual causes include anoxia (as by blockage of arterial supply), physical agents (trauma, heat, cold, radiant energy), chemical agents (corrosives, poisons), and biologic agents (pathogenic bacteria, viruses, fungi, protozoa).

Irreversible cell injury appears to be due to a significant cell membrane injury, which permits an influx of Ca^{+2}. The excessive accumulation of Ca^{+2} in the cytosol and mitochondria impairs cellular functions, and cell death results.

Coagulation necrosis occurs characteristically in the myocardium, lung, kidney, and spleen as a result of the sudden, complete blockage of a branch of the arterial tree which results in local ischemia. As a consequence of anoxia, the affected cells of the organ die and cytoplasmic and intracellular proteins become denatured or coagulated. Microscopically, faint outlines of tissue structure can be recognized in the area of necrosis. The nuclei of dead cells are pyknotic or absent. The area of necrosis is sharply delimited from the surrounding normal tissue.

Liquefaction necrosis occurs characteristically in the brain or spinal cord as a result of the sudden, complete blockage of an arterial branch and rapid enzymatic dissolution of lipids. The precise cause of the liquefaction is not known. Liquefaction necrosis also occurs in abscesses in any organ or tissue, as a result of the invasion of the tissues by pyogenic bacteria and the consequent outpouring of leukocytes. From these leukocytes, lytic lysosomal enzymes are released into the tissues, and the mass of dead cells is liquefied.

Caseation necrosis occurs as a result of infection by Mycobacterium tuberculosis and Histoplasma capsulatum. The affected tissues are converted to granular yellow, crumbly, friable material resembling cheese. Microscopically, the underlying tissue is often unrecognizable and is replaced by granular eosinophilic material.

Fibrinoid necrosis occurs characteristically in the walls of small arteries of people with malignant hypertension. It also occurs in vessel walls and fibrous connective tissues, as in polyarteritis nodosa due to immunologic injury. The fibrillar structure which normally gives a layered pattern to the tissue is replaced by a granular smudgy material which stains intensely with eosin.

Fat necrosis occurs in adipose tissue and may be a result of trauma, bacterial invasion, or chemical injury. As a result of lipase action, there is hydrolysis of neutral fat, and white chalky deposits of calcium soaps are formed in the tissues. In the omentum and mesentery, fat necrosis usually means chemical injury due to the escape of pancreatic lipase into the peritoneal cavity as a result of acute pancreatitis. Microscopically, the fat appears as sheets of round cells with a granular cytoplasm which stains basophilically because of the calcium.

Items 16-21

In Items 16-21, match each disorder with the type of hemorrhage which typically occurs with it.

> (A) ecchymosis
> (B) epistaxis
> (C) hematemesis
> (D) hemoptysis
> (E) melena
> (F) metrorrhagia
> (G) petechiae

16. battered child syndrome

17. duodenal ulcer

18. fractured nose

19. portal hypertension

20. thrombocytopenia

21. tuberculosis of lung

ANSWERS AND TUTORIAL ON ITEMS 16-21

The answers are: **16-A; 17-E; 18-B; 19-C; 20-G; 21-D**. Hemorrhage is the escape of blood from a vessel incident to a mechanical defect in the vascular or cardiac wall. Definitions relating to hemorrhage are:

> Ecchymosis. A blotchy, purplish hemorrhage into the subcutaneous tissues due to leakage from venules; a bruise. Typically due to blunt trauma.

8

Epistaxis. A hemorrhage from the nose.

Hematemesis. The presence of a significant amount of blood in vomitus, due to a ruptured esophageal varix secondary to portal hypertension.

Hematoma. A localized mass of blood, usually clotted, within a tissue.

Hemoptysis. The presence of blood in the sputum. Common causes are bronchiectasis and pulmonary tuberculosis.

Hemostasis. The stopping of blood flow from the vascular tree.

Melena. The presence of dark, digested blood in the feces. A bleeding duodenal ulcer is a common cause.

Menorrhagia. Excessive endometrial bleeding during a menstrual period.

Metrorrhagia. Irregular endometrial bleeding between menstrual periods.

Petechia. A tiny hemorrhage due to leakage from a capillary or venule. It is often associated with thrombocytopenia.

The causes of hemorrhage include injury, infection, or ulceration of a blood vessel wall; atherosclerosis, in which the arterial wall becomes brittle; rupture of an aneurysm (a bulge in a vessel wall); purpuras (bleeding diseases in which small hemorrhages occur in the skin and mucosa); leukemia, because of the suppression of platelet formation; avitaminosis K, because of the deficiency of prothrombin formation; scurvy (avitaminosis C), because of fragility of the vessel walls; certain poisons and bacterial toxins; and hypoxia.

When even a large amount of blood is lost over a long period of time, as in chronically bleeding hemorrhoids, the body is able to compensate by increasing the activity of the bone marrow to replace the shed erythrocytes. When blood loss outstrips replacement, anemia ensues.

Hemorrhage into the gastrointestinal tract, abdominal cavity, or retroperitoneal region has the same effect as external hemorrhage. Pleural or pericardial hemorrhage may compress the lungs or heart (cardiac tamponade). Cerebral hemorrhage infiltrates the adjacent brain substance and destroys it.

Items 22-25

A 40 year-old woman with mitral stenosis from rheumatic heart disease went into intractable left ventricular failure and died. A photomicrograph of a section of lung at autopsy is shown in Figure 1.3.

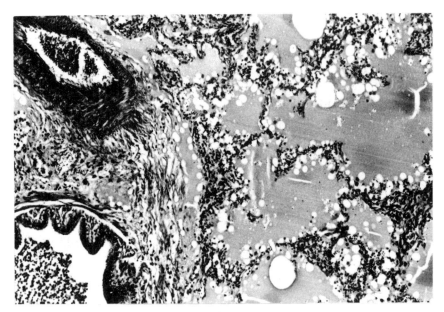

Figure 1.3

22.   The likeliest diagnosis is

    (A)   bronchopneumonia
    (B)   congestion and edema
    (C)   infarction
    (D)   lobar pneumonia
    (E)   lymphedema

23.   In a patient with chronic right ventricular failure, the usual pathologic change which occurs in the liver is

    (A)   acute inflammation
    (B)   congestion
    (C)   edema
    (D)   hemorrhage
    (E)   infarction

24.   The basic causes of edema include all of the following **EXCEPT**:

    (A)   increased capillary blood pressure
    (B)   increased permeability of capillaries and venules
    (C)   increased plasma osmotic pressure
    (D)   obstruction of lymph flow
    (E)   sodium retention by the kidneys

25.   A teenage boy has episodes of swelling of the upper lip and abdominal pain. There is a family history of angioneurotic edema. The defect underlying the episodes is

    (A)   abnormal sensitivity to histamine
    (B)   deficiency of $C'1$ esterase inhibitor
    (C)   excessive degranulation of mast cells by $C'5a$
    (D)   hypersensitivity to kinins
    (E)   membrane damage by $C'56789$

ANSWERS AND TUTORIAL ON ITEMS 22-25

The answers are: **22-B; 23-B; 24-C; 25-B**.

The photomicrograph in Figure 1.3 shows hyperemia of the pulmonary capillaries and small arteries, together with coagulated transudate in the alveolar spaces. These changes are characteristic of congestion and edema. Increased plasma osmotic pressure is not a cause of edema because it would tend to hold water within blood vessels.

In patients with congestive heart failure, when the right heart becomes involved, back-pressure in the inferior vena cava and hepatic vein leads to congestion within the hepatic sinusoids.

Hyperemia (congestion) is the presence of an abnormally increased amount of blood within the finer vessels of a tissue. Active hyperemia is a dynamic congestion due to an increased flow of arterial blood to a part. It results from the dilatation of arterioles, as in muscles during exercise, flushing of the face, or foci of acute inflammation.

Passive congestion results from obstruction or hindrance to the outflow of venous blood from a part. It may be general (as in cardiac failure) or local. The causes of passive congestion include ineffective cardiac action (congestive heart failure); pressure of a mass or scar tissue on a vein; pregnancy (by pressure on pelvic veins); venous thrombosis; twisting of the intestinal mesentery or a cyst pedicle with resultant venous compression; and compression of a vein by a tight bandage, tourniquet, or ligature.

Edema is a dynamic pathologic process characterized by the accumulation of an abnormal amount of fluid in the cells, intercellular spaces, and/or cavities of the body due to conditions which upset the mechanisms of fluid balance or which interfere with normal lymph flow.

Definitions relating to edema are:

Anasarca. Edema of the body as a whole.

Ascites. A collection of edema fluid in the peritoneal cavity.

Exudate. Edema fluid with a specific gravity above 1.015 and a protein level above 3 percent. It occurs in acute inflammations as a result of increased blood-tissue barrier permeability.

Transudate. Edema fluid with a specific gravity below 1.015 and a protein content below 3 percent. It results from increased capillary hydrostatic pressure with normal permeability.

The basic causes of edema are obstruction to lymph flow (lymphedema), abnormal permeability of capillaries and venules, increased capillary blood pressure, decreased plasma colloidal osmotic pressure, decreased extravascular tissue pressure, and excessive sodium ion retention by the kidneys.

Lymphedema is an increase of tissue fluid resulting from obstruction of the lymph flow from an area. Lymphatic blockage may be due to malignant neoplastic cells within lymph channels or nodes, parasites (especially filaria) within lymph channels, chronic inflammation (by causing scar tissue to form about lymph channels), or removal of a lymph node group by surgery. The edema is localized to the tissues normally drained by the obstructed lymph channels.

Angioneurotic edema is an intermittent and rapidly developing local swelling of the skin, lips, respiratory mucosa, stomach, and intestines. In the sporadic type, the swelling results from a hypersensitivity reaction. The uncommon hereditary type is transmitted as an autosomal dominant. Patients with the hereditary angioneurotic edema have a deficiency of the inhibitor of activated first component of complement (C'1 esterase inhibitor). This leads to excessive production of C'2-kinin, which causes increased vascular permeability.

Items 26-38

26. The formation of a coagulum of blood in an artery or vein during life is

    (A) congestion
    (B) embolism
    (C) hemorrhage
    (D) infarction
    (E) thrombosis

27. Platelet aggregation at the site of blood vessel injury is initiated by

    (A) activation of Hageman factor
    (B) contact of platelets with subendothelial collagen
    (C) lysosomal enzymes from neutrophils
    (D) release of tissue thromboplastin
    (E) thrombin

12

28.   Causes of increased tendency to thrombosis include all of the following **EXCEPT**:

   (A)   aspirin abuse
   (B)   atherosclerosis
   (C)   increased blood viscosity
   (D)   pancreatic carcinoma
   (E)   use of an intravascular catheter

29.   When a left ventricular mural thrombus develops, infarction may result in all of the following **EXCEPT**:

   (A)   cerebrum
   (B)   kidneys
   (C)   lungs
   (D)   small intestine
   (E)   spleen

In Items 30-33, match each disorder with the type of embolism typically associated with it.

   (A)   air embolism
   (B)   fat embolism
   (C)   paradoxical embolism
   (D)   septic embolism
   (E)   talc embolism

30.   acute bacterial endocarditis

31.   fracture of bone

32.   interventricular septal defect

33.   intravenous drug use

An elderly woman, bedridden because of congestive heart failure, complained of sudden, severe chest pain. She died within a few minutes. A photograph of the lungs at autopsy is shown in Figure 1.4.

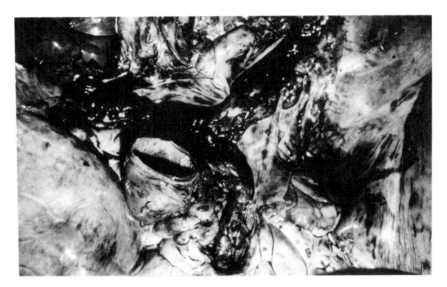

Figure 1.4

34. The likeliest cause of death in this case is

   (A)   bronchopneumonia
   (B)   hemorrhagic infarction of lungs
   (C)   congestion and edema of lungs
   (D)   pulmonary embolism
   (E)   pulmonary arterial thrombosis

35. The impaction of a coagulum of blood in a vessel at a point beyond which it cannot pass is

   (A)   congestion
   (B)   embolism
   (C)   hemorrhage
   (D)   infarction
   (E)   thrombosis

14

A month before death, a 65 year-old man suffered sharp costovertebral angle pain and had an episode of hematuria. A photograph of the involved kidney is shown in Figure 1.5.

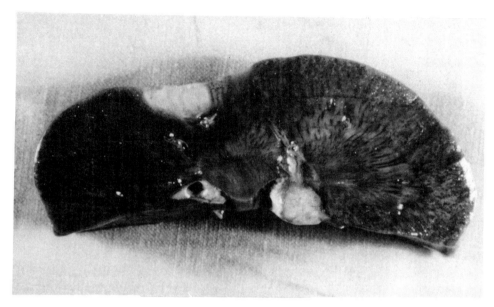

Figure 1.5

36.   The likeliest diagnosis in this kidney is

    (A)   abscess
    (B)   adenoma
    (C)   carcinoma
    (D)   hematoma
    (E)   infarct

37.   Hemorrhagic infarction characteristically occurs in the

    (A)   kidney
    (B)   liver
    (C)   lungs
    (D)   myocardium
    (E)   pancreas

38. In embolism to a branch of the splenic artery, the origin of the embolus may be any of the following **EXCEPT**:

(A) complicated atheromatous plaque in thoracic aorta
(B) mural thrombus in left ventricle
(C) thrombus in abdominal aortic aneurysm
(D) thrombus in left atrial appendage
(E) thrombus in calf vein with patent foramen ovale

ANSWERS AND TUTORIAL ON ITEMS 26-38

The answers are: **26-E; 27-B; 28-A; 29-C; 30-D; 31-B; 32-C; 33-E; 34-D; 35-B; 36-E; 37-C; 38-C**.

Formation of a coagulum of blood in a vessel during life is thrombosis, and the coagulum is a thrombus. The process is often initiated by contact of platelets with subendothelial collagen. Platelets release ADP which causes platelet aggregation. The coagulation mechanism is triggered, and thrombosis results.

The photograph in Item 34 shows a large embolus blocking the main pulmonary arteries. Such an embolus usually originates as a thrombus in a vein of the lower leg, breaking off to impact in the pulmonary circulation. This sequence of events is common in bed-ridden patients.

The photograph in Item 36 shows a roughly wedge-shaped pale subcapsular focus of old infarction in the kidney. It may have resulted from thrombosis in or embolism to a renal arterial branch supplying the infarcted zone. This infarct is pale (anemic). Hemorrhagic infarcts usually occur in soft organs, such as the lungs or intestine. Infarcts due to venous occlusion are often hemorrhagic.

Splenic arterial embolism cannot be due to a thrombus from an abdominal aortic aneurysm because the abdominal aorta is distal to the splenic circulation.

The basic causes of thrombosis are injury, inflammation, or degeneration of a blood vessel wall; slowing, stasis, or eddying of the blood flow; and increased coagulability of the blood.

Blood vessel injury may be due to mechanical trauma, such as fractures and bullet or knife wounds; ligation or clamping during surgery, burns; and cold. Blood vessel inflammation occurs in thrombophlebitis, in which clotting occurs within veins. Arterial degeneration occurs as atherosclerosis, with hyalin and lipid deposits and calcification in the intima. Thrombi frequently form on atherosclerotic plaques at the zone of intimal degeneration.

Slowing or eddying of the blood in an auricular appendage, such as in auricular fibrillation, often leads to thrombosis. Such a thrombus as well as a mural one may become pedunculated and act as a ball-valve thrombus. Thrombosis may also occur in an aneurysmal sac due to eddying within the bulged-out portion of the vessel. Thrombosis occurring without a precedent alteration in a vein wall is phlebothrombosis and is usually due to slowing or stasis of the blood within the vein. Such thrombosis usually originates in the pockets behind valve cusps in lower extremity veins. Pressure of a space-occupying mass or of a pregnant uterus on veins produces slowing of the venous flow distally, and thrombosis sometimes follows. The general circulatory slowing in congestive heart failure, together with the inactivity of the cardiac patient, is accompanied by a tendency to venous thrombosis.

Increased coagulability of the blood is caused by the release of tissue thromboplastin or other procoagulants in disseminated intravascular coagulation. A tendency to thrombosis may also be present in conditions characterized by increased blood viscosity due to a striking increase in the number of cells, such as chronic leukemia and polycythemia. A migratory phlebothrombosis complicates some cases of malignant neoplasm, especially pancreatic carcinoma, due to increased coagulability of the blood.

Occlusion of a vein may produce stasis in the area drained, causing passive hyperemia or even necrosis of the involved tissues. Occlusion of an artery causes ischemia of the tissue supplied. Unless collateral circulation is present and adequate, infarction will follow. If the thrombus becomes detached and free in the circulation, it is an embolus. Some thrombi are removed by lysis. If a thrombus remains attached and the patient survives, it becomes organized from the lining of the vessel. Capillaries bud into the thrombotic mass, fibroblasts proliferate, and gradually the thrombus is replaced. New vascular channels develop through it (recanalization), or the mass becomes fibrous.

Embolism is the lodging of an embolus in a blood vessel at a point beyond which it cannot pass. An embolus is a foreign substance such as a thrombus or fragments of a thrombus, tissue cells, clumps of bacteria, parasites, bone marrow, amniotic fluid, globules of fat, or bubbles of gas carried in the bloodstream. Fragments of or entire thrombi are by far the most common type of emboli. Venous emboli originate in the peripheral veins and almost always lodge in a pulmonary artery, producing infarction of a lung, or sudden death in cases of massive embolism.

In over 90 percent of the cases, pulmonary emboli arise in veins of the lower extremities, especially the deep calf veins. Small or large thrombi break off from a site of phlebothrombosis and are carried in the venous bloodstream up the inferior vena cava and though the right side of the heart into the pulmonary arterial circulation, where they impact. When a large embolus is suddenly jammed into the main pulmonary artery or is impacted astride the bifurcation to block both great pulmonary trunks (saddle embolus), the pulmonary circulation is completely obstructed and an enormous strain is immediately placed on the right ventricle. There is a rapid rise in the pulmonary arterial pressure proximal to the block, and the right ventricle and atrium become dilated (acute cor pulmonale). Death may ensue within a few minutes due to the failure of venous return to the left side of the heart. A shower of small emboli which lodge in numerous pulmonary arterial branches may produce similar results.

Arterial emboli originate from the left side of the heart, an aneurysmal sac, an atheromatous plaque on a large arterial trunk, or rarely, the pulmonary veins. The effects of arterial emboli depend on the size and nature of the embolus, the organ involved, and the state of collateral circulation. If collateral circulation is absent or deficient, an embolus of any size will produce infarction in the heart, brain, spleen, intestine, kidney, or an extremity.

Paradoxical embolism results when a venous embolus enters the arterial circulation through a patent foramen ovale or other cardiac septal defect.

Septic embolism is the lodgement of infected foreign material in a blood vessel. Masses of bacteria, usually within a septic embolus, are carried in the bloodstream. Septic infarcts or abscesses are produced where the emboli lodge. In some cases, necrosis of the artery in which the infected embolus lodges leads to thinning and outpouching of the wall (mycotic aneurysm).

Neutral fats from injured tissue or the bone marrow, or injected fats and oils, may act as fat emboli, obstructing capillaries in the lungs, brain, and elsewhere. Most cases follow fractures or other trauma to fat. Fat embolism also occurs in cases of fatty liver in acute and chronic alcoholism, carbon tetrachloride poisoning, diabetes mellitus, and decompression sickness.

Talc, cellulose, and cornstarch embolism in the pulmonary circulation occurs in addicts who inject oral drug preparations intravenously. The starch and talc are used as fillers for drugs, such as amphetamines and barbiturates, or as adulterants with heroin. In persons who inject drugs, foreign-body granulomas that consist of filler granules, macrophages, and epithelioid and multinucleated giant cells develop in and around the walls of small pulmonary arteries. Thrombi develop within the lumina of these vessels. Extensive occlusion of the pulmonary arterial tree may occur with resultant pulmonary hypertension and cor pulmonale.

Infarction is the production of an infarct, a local focus of necrosis resulting from vascular obstruction. When an artery is occluded suddenly, cell death occurs in the tissues supplied by it. The vessels and capillaries deprived of blood later dilate and fill with blood from surrounding anastomoses. A fresh infarct is therefore dark and congested. In soft organs, such as the lungs and intestines, hemorrhagic infarcts occur. In a firm organ, such as the kidney, swelling of parenchymal cells presses the blood out of small vessels so that a pale (anemic) infarct occurs.

A man with poor dentition and oral hygiene developed chills and fever. A chest film revealed a small, round opacity in the RLL. A photomicrograph of the lesion from a segmental resection is shown in Figure 1.6.

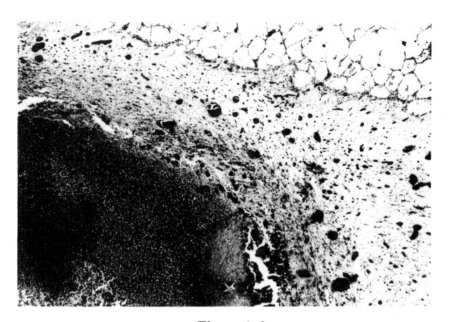

Figure 1.6

39.   The likeliest diagnosis is

(A)   abscess
(B)   bronchopneumonia
(C)   carcinoma
(D)   infarct
(E)   tuberculosis

40.   The type of necrosis in the lesion shown above is

(A)   caseation
(B)   coagulation
(C)   fibrinoid
(D)   hemorrhagic
(E)   liquefaction

41. The cause of the type of necrosis shown above is

    (A)   arterial occlusion by an embolus
    (B)   bacterial toxins
    (C)   cell-mediated immune reaction
    (D)   lysosomal enzymes from neutrophils
    (E)   outgrowth of blood supply by malignant cells

42. The process by which inflammatory cells are positively attracted to a focus of tissue injury is

    (A)   anaphylaxis
    (B)   chemotaxis
    (C)   complement fixation
    (D)   migration
    (E)   phagocytosis

43. Digestion of foreign material by a neutrophil or macrophage during phagocytosis is mainly due to

    (A)   complement
    (B)   hydrogen peroxide
    (C)   kinins
    (D)   lysosomal enzymes
    (E)   thrombin

44. A major cause of pain in foci of acute inflammation is

    (A)   bradykinin
    (B)   complement
    (C)   histamine
    (D)   hydrogen peroxide
    (E)   superoxide

45. A 1 year-old boy had frequent infections due to Staphylococcus aureus. NADPH oxidase activity in his neutrophils was absent, and H_2O_2 was not formed. The most likely diagnosis is

    (A)   Chediak-Higashi syndrome
    (B)   chronic granulomatous disease
    (C)   Job's syndrome
    (D)   lazy leukocyte syndrome
    (E)   myeloperoxidase deficiency

46. Granulomatous inflammation is characteristic of all of the following **EXCEPT**:

   (A) berylliosis
   (B) foreign body reaction
   (C) fungus infections
   (D) leprosy
   (E) pertussis

47. Foci of granulomatous inflammation show all of the following **EXCEPT**:

   (A) eosinophils
   (B) epithelioid cells
   (C) fibrosis
   (D) lymphocytes
   (E) multinucleated giant cells

48. A large scar due to excessive collagen formation is a

   (A) callus
   (B) cicatrix
   (C) keloid
   (D) proud flesh
   (E) suture granuloma

49. Cells which are capable of regeneration to replace cells of the same type destroyed by injury include all of the following **EXCEPT**:

   (A) epidermis
   (B) hepatocytes
   (C) intestinal epithelium
   (D) myocardial fibers
   (E) renal tubular epithelium

50. Factors which delay or prevent wound healing include all of the following **EXCEPT**:

   (A) ionizing radiation
   (B) protein deficiency
   (C) ultraviolet light
   (D) vitamin C deficiency
   (E) zinc deficiency

ANSWERS AND TUTORIAL ON ITEMS 39-50

The answers are: **39-A; 40-E; 41-D; 42-B; 43-D; 44-A; 45-B; 46-E; 47-A; 48-C; 49-D; 50-C**.

The photomicrograph in Item 39 shows a focus of lung tissue destruction due to liquefaction necrosis. This is caused by release of lytic lysosomal enzymes from dead neutrophils in the lung abscess. The abscess is walled off by a collagenous membrane. Lung abscess due to anaerobic bacteria from the mouth is associated with poor dentition and oral hygiene due to inhalation. An abscess is a localized collection of pus in a tissue. It is filled with viable and dead phagocytes and bacteria.

The local reaction of tissues to an injurious agent is inflammation. When a tissue is inoculated with a small quantity of a living culture of virulent bacteria, a series of vascular changes takes place, sometimes beginning with a transient constriction of blood vessels. Soon the arterioles dilate, causing a speeding of blood flow. Next, venules and then capillaries dilate, resulting in hyperemia, with stagnation of the circulation. As the vessels dilate and the flow of blood slows, the vessel walls become more permeable. Leukocytes and plasma move out of vessels into the connective tissues, forming the inflammatory exudate. Subsequent developments depend chiefly upon the amount of tissue destroyed. If tissue destruction is minimal, the dead cells are removed, hyperemia subsides, and the tissues return almost to normal, leaving no scar. If there is extensive destruction of tissue, great numbers of leukocytes come into the area and release their lytic enzymes. The central portion of the affected tissues liquefies, forming an abscess, or, if at a surface, an ulcer. If bacterial multiplication gets ahead of the host's response, the infection may spread to adjacent parts, and the process may end with the death of the host due to systemic effects of the infection.

The vascular response in acute inflammation is biphasic. The early phase lasting a few minutes is mediated by histamine released locally from tissue mast cells. Vasodilation and increased endothelial permeability are produced by histamine. The delayed and sustained phase, which becomes maximal in 3-4 hours, is mediated mainly by kinins. Following tissue injury, kinins incite vascular dilatation, increased vascular permeability, and emigration of leukocytes. Bradykinin is a nine amino acid peptide which, when injected locally, causes severe pain and tissue changes which closely simulate those occurring naturally in an acute inflammation. Prostaglandins PGE and PGI_2 cause vasodilation and pain synergistically with bradykinin in foci of inflammation. These actions are inhibited by aspirin and other nonsteroidal anti-inflammatory agents. Leukotrienes C, D, and E (slow reacting substance, SRS) cause a short-lived vasoconstriction, especially of arterioles, followed by increased vascular permeability.

In the focus of acute inflammation leukocytes escape from the bloodstream into the affected tissues. First the cells move out of the axial stream and adhere to the vascular lining (margination). Divalent cations, especially Ca^{+2}, play a key role in mediating leukocyte sticking. As the venules dilate, endothelial cells lining these vessels are pulled apart, exposing the underlying basement membrane to the leukocytes. These cells then emigrate into the perivascular connective tissues, passing between endothelial cells and through the basement membrane. Cells are attracted to the area of tissue injury by a positive force known as chemotaxis. Chemoattractants include C'5a, leukotriene B4, and bacterial soluble products.

As the leukocytes move into the area of tissue injury, they provide an additional source of kinins. Plasma always seeps out of the vessels along with leukocytes. This exudation of leukocytes and plasma separates the fixed tissues of the affected part and leads to swelling (inflammatory edema). Plasma brings with it its various ingredients such as the plasma proteins, including in some instances, specific antibodies capable of acting against the infectious agents or neutralizing its toxins.

The polymorphonuclear leukocyte (PMN) (neutrophil) is particularly important in acute inflammation. The PMNs contain lysosomes. These granules contain several potent lytic enzymes which make it possible for these cells to destroy many types of bacteria and to liquefy the cell fragments resulting from tissue injury. The formation of hydrogen peroxide within neutrophils contributes to the bactericidal effect of these cells, as does the presence of superoxide, myeloperoxidase, and halide ions, especially OCl^-.

Meanwhile, other changes have occurred in the area of injury. The blood in the small vessels, already stagnant from vasodilatation, becomes more viscous. Thrombosis of small vessels commonly occurs. Strands of fibrin also form in tissue interstices as the result of the interaction of the coagulation-prompting factors present in the exudate. The fibrin web tends to block the movement of tissue fluids, thereby localizing the bacterial agent in the case of staphylococcal infections. In streptococcal infections, fibrinolytic enzymes are active in the exudate, and there is less tendency for the infection to remain localized. A spreading infection (cellulitis) is common.

The cardinal signs of inflammation have been known for centuries. Calor (heat) and rubor (redness) are manifestations of the active hyperemia in the affected part. Tumor (swelling) is due chiefly to the accumulation of the inflammatory exudate but also to hyperemia. Dolor (pain) and functio laesa (disturbed function) are due to a combination of factors including the stimulation of sensory nerve endings as the exudate stretches the tissues, and the direct effect of kinins. Fever is due to resetting of the hypothalamic thermoregulator by endogenous pyrogens [interleukin-1, tumor necrosis factor (TNF), and prostaglandins] released from macrophages and neutrophils. Leukocytosis results from the release of colony stimulating factor from macrophages.

In chronic inflammation, the injurious agent acts over a longer period of time but is less damaging than in the examples of acute inflammation. In such cases, tissue destruction, hyperemia, and exudation may be minimal or non-existent, lymphocytes and macrophages predominate in the exudate, and fibrous tissue proliferation may be marked.

A special form of chronic inflammation is seen in response to tissue invasion by Mycobacterium tuberculosis. Macrophages and multinucleated giant cells accumulate about the organisms, and fibrous tissue forms about these small focal lesions or tubercles. This combination of macrophages and fibrosis is granulomatous inflammation. Epithelioid cells and multinucleated Langhans giant cells are present. The former are derived from macrophages and the latter by cytoplasmic fusion of macrophages. These lesions may heal by scarring and become calcified, or they may undergo caseation necrosis. Similar focal collections of macrophages without caseation may be seen in certain other diseases (fungus infections, leprosy, syphilis, sarcoid, brucellosis); these focal lesions are often spoken of as tuberculoid granulomas. Beryllium, when inhaled into the lung or deposited in a wound, may incite a similar granulomatous inflammation.

Another form of chronic inflammation is seen as a reaction to foreign material in the tissues. Usually the material is organic matter, such as vegetable fibers or hair, but a similar reaction occurs with suture material. Macrophages are attracted to the area, and a number of them, perhaps a dozen or even as many as 50, fuse, resulting in a multinucleated giant cell. These cells engulf the foreign matter. Lymphocytes and fibrous tissue formation are always seen in conjunction with the giant cells.

The special role of leukocytes is emphasized by the peculiar susceptibility to infection of those individuals whose leukocytes are reduced in number or impaired in quality. Patients with marked leukopenia are very susceptible to infections. Patients who receive cancer chemotherapy may show a leukocyte count of 1,000/mm^3 as a result of the cytotoxic effect of the drug on leukocyte precursors in the bone marrow. These patients often develop opportunistic infections - bacterial, fungal, or viral - to which they succumb. In such cases, the inflammatory exudate may contain fewer leukocytes than is usual with the organism in question, making microscopic diagnosis difficult.

There are many instances in which leukocytes are present in normal numbers but are somehow impaired in quality. Since leukocyte dysfunctions are usually caused by hereditary disorders, the effects are manifest in infancy or early childhood as an unusual susceptibility to infection. These dysfunctions include defective chemotaxis and migration related to deficiency or inhibition of complement components; failure of recognition related to absence of opsonization of bacteria as a result of a lack of activation of C'3; a disorder of degranulation caused by the absence of NADPH oxidase and failure of peroxidation (formation of hydrogen peroxide), which usually occurs as an X-chromosome-linked chronic granulomatous disease of young males.

Chediak-Higashi syndrome is inherited as an autosomal recessive trait. The disease appears to be a generalized abnormality of unit membrane-bound organelles, such as lysosomes. The syndrome becomes clinically apparent at from one to eight years of age with partial albinism, photophobia, lymphadenopathy, hepatosplenomegaly, and decreased resistance to infections. The last is caused by decreased bactericidal activity of neutrophils. This is due to decreased chemotactic responsiveness and phagocytic activity. Death typically occurs by the age of 10 years due to infection or development of a malignant lymphoma. Large cytoplasmic granules are present in leukocytes.

Job's syndrome occurs in light-skinned, red-haired girls. There is defective neutrophilic chemotactic response. The patients have repeated suppurative lymphadenitis and staphylococcal abscesses without signs of inflammation. Serum levels of immunoglobulin E (IgE) are markedly elevated.

Inflammation and healing should be looked upon as two parts of a single vital function, the physiologic response to tissue injury, the objective of which is restoration of normal structure and function. Perfect restoration of function is dependent upon the replacement of lost cells by like cells (regeneration), and the orderly arrangement of these new cells in relation to preexisting cells so that intercellular functions are restored. This is not possible in all tissues. Repair, i.e., filling in of a wound or tissue defect, may restore lost tissue mass, but this is not the same as regeneration. Certain cell strains (epidermis, intestinal epithelium, and hematopoietic cells) continue to undergo cell division throughout life (intermitotic cells), whereas others (fixed postmitotic cells, such as neurons, skeletal muscle, and cardiac muscle) do not. This difference in reproductive capability is apparently due to the presence or absence of intermitotic cells in adult tissues. Tissues which have them are able to regenerate after injury; tissues which lack them cannot. Intermediate between these two extremes are reverting postmitotic cells, such as hepatocytes, renal tubular epithelial cells, and connective tissues in general. Tissues composed of these cells normally contain few intermitotic cells, but when tissue is lost, surviving cells are capable of a rapid increase in the rate of cell division.

All wounds heal in roughly the same way: new cells are formed from preexisting cells and fill in the area of tissue loss, receiving support and nourishment from connective tissue and blood vessels as they grow. Small wounds heal quickly, large wounds slowly. A clean, dry surgical wound heals rapidly by primary union. By contrast, a gaping wound must fill in by granulation before the surface epithelium can cover it over. Healing has then occurred by secondary union.

Collagen is the chief constituent of scar tissue. Tropocollagen is synthesized by myofibroblasts and extruded into the extracellular space, where it polymerizes to form the banded collagen fibrils. These fibrils then arrange themselves parallel to each other to form an orderly sheet. As collagen ages, the bonds between fibrils continue to grow stronger. Thus, the healed wound continues to gain tensile strength. A large scar caused by excessive collagen formation is a keloid.

The following systemic factors promote wound healing; youth (wound healing is a slower process in the elderly person), warmth, ultra-violet light, and good nutrition, particularly adequate reserves of protein. The following systemic factors delay or prevent wound healing; vitamin C or zinc deficiency, protein starvation, prolonged therapy with steroids (by suppressing the vascular phase of inflammation), and ionizing radiation. Local factors which inhibit wound healing include presence of foreign matter, poor blood supply, and persistence of infection.

Items 51-60

A 65 year-old cigarette smoker developed worsening of his usual cough, together with weight loss and hemoptysis. A pneumonectomy was performed. A photograph of the gross surgical specimen is shown in Figure 1.7.

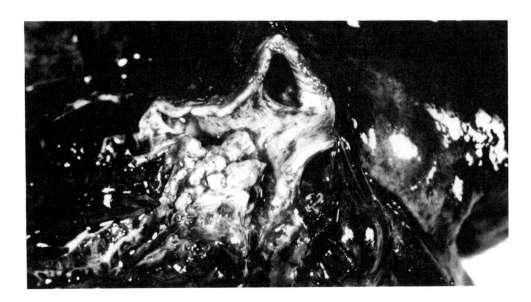

Figure 1.7

51.   The likeliest diagnosis is

(A)   adenoma
(B)   bronchiectasis
(C)   metastatic carcinoma
(D)   primary carcinoma
(E)   sarcoma

52.   A carcinoma is a malignant neoplasm of

(A)   connective tissue cells
(B)   epithelial cells
(C)   lymphocytes
(D)   muscle fibers
(E)   neurons

53. The phenomenon which most definitely indicates that a neoplasm is malignant is

   (A) autonomous cell proliferation
   (B) central necrosis
   (C) lack of encapsulation
   (D) metastasis
   (E) painfulness

54. All the following chemicals are carcinogens **EXCEPT**:

   (A) asbestos
   (B) aspartame
   (C) benzpyrene
   (D) methylcholanthrene
   (E) vinyl chloride

55. All of the following are features of benign neoplasms **EXCEPT**:

   (A) autonomous growth
   (B) circumscription
   (C) encapsulation
   (D) invasion
   (E) resemblance of tumor cells to normal

In Items 56-59, match each type of cancer with the cause known or strongly suspected to be associated with it.

   (A) aniline dyes
   (B) aflatoxin
   (C) Epstein-Barr virus
   (D) nitrates
   (E) papilloma virus

56. cervical carcinoma

57. hepatocarcinoma

58. Burkitt's lymphoma

59. urinary bladder carcinoma

60. Increased incidences of cancer are associated with all of the following **EXCEPT**:

   (A)   cancer chemotherapeutic drugs
   (B)   chromosomal defects
   (C)   immunodeficiency
   (D)   infrared radiation
   (E)   ultraviolet radiation

ANSWERS AND TUTORIAL ON ITEMS 51-60

The answers are: **51-D; 52-B; 53-D; 54-B; 55-D; 56-E; 57-B; 58-C; 59-A; 60-D**.

> The photograph in Item 51 shows an irregular, poorly outlined mass arising in a large bronchus and invading the adjacent lung parenchyma. These features are characteristic of a malignant neoplasm, in this case most likely a primary bronchogenic carcinoma. Metastatic carcinoma typically shows multiple foci in the lungs. Carcinomas are malignant neoplasms arising from epithelial cells. Sarcomas are cancers arising in connective tissue cells. The most definitive indicator of malignancy in a tumor is the development of a metastasis.

A neoplasm is a focal autonomous new growth of cells which has no useful function. Neoplasia is the process of development of neoplasms (tumors).

Benign neoplasms do not invade adjacent tissue nor spread to distant sites and are the cause of localized effects. In contrast, malignant tumors invade normal tissue, spread elsewhere in the body, and cause death by local and disseminated effects. Benign tumors are much more common than malignant tumors and tend to arise at an earlier age and to enlarge at a slower rate. Benign tumors are cured by total excision, whereas malignant tumors are often incurable because of spread outside the resectable region.

Grossly, benign neoplasms are characterized by sharply circumscribed margins that are often encapsulated, by central portions that tend to remain solid and viable, and by a texture that is uniformly soft or resilient. The microscopic feature is the resemblance of benign tumor cells to normal cells so that while the tissue pattern is altered and ordinarily easily distinguished from normal, the individual cells are often not.

Malignant neoplasms (cancers) are characterized grossly by serrated margins due to irregular invasion of adjacent tissues, by foci of necrosis in their centers, and sometimes by a hard consistency. Microscopically, they are characterized by a pronounced distortion of cell pattern. The most conspicuous changes are variations in cell size and shape; increase in nuclear size and nucleocytoplasmic ratio; increased nuclear staining (hyperchromatism); and increased numbers of mitotic figures, some of which are abnormal. Malignancy often involves appearance of discrete tumor nodules in parts of the body separated from the primary site. This phenomenon (metastasis) is due to the detachment of tumor cells from the site of origin and their transport in the lymph or blood streams to other tissues, especially lymph nodes, liver, and lungs. While this phenomenon is proof of malignancy, the absence of metastasis does not establish benign behavior.

Certain biochemical changes are also utilized for the diagnosis of cancer. Choriocarcinoma is accompanied by a high concentration of chorionic gonadotrophin in the serum, and the decline of this substance in the blood after the removal of the uterus is indicative of cure, while persistence of an elevated blood level is suggestive of metastatic disease. Normal cells and malignant epithelial tumors of the prostate produce acid phosphatase which usually escapes in the pathway of secretions of the gland through the urethra. With cancerous invasion of paraprostatic tissue, and especially with metastasis to bone, the circulating level undergoes a sharp rise and is accordingly useful in the diagnosis of metastatic disease from this site. Prostate specific antigen (PSA) is a more specific screening test, being elevated in prostatic carcinoma. Additional examples are the presence of significant amounts of 5-hydroxytryptamine (serotonin) in the blood in cases of metastatic carcinoid, calcitonin in medullary thyroid carcinoma, α-fetoprotein in hepatocarcinoma, and carcinoembryonic antigen (CEA) in colon carcinoma.

Some neoplasms produce potent clinical manifestations by excessive secretion of hormones. Islet cell adenoma or carcinoma may cause severe hypoglycemia by insulin secretion, and hypertension may result from release of large amounts of catecholamines from a pheochromocytoma of the adrenal medulla. A paraneoplastic syndrome occurs when neoplastic cells produce a hormone not normally secreted by the cells of origin. Anaplastic bronchogenic carcinoma sometimes elaborates significant amounts of adrenocorticotrophic hormone, antidiuretic hormone, or parathormone with resultant endocrine effects.

The ultimate cause of malignant transformation in a cell or group of cells is unknown. It appears to be an alteration in nuclear DNA which produces a modification of gene expression, either as the result of a random mutation or the effect of a carcinogenic agent. Once induced, malignant transformation is a hereditably transmissible cellular change characterized by escape from normal growth controls; increased capacity for growth; cell membrane alterations and decreased adherence between cells which lead to a loosening of intercellular bonds; loss of contact inhibition between adjacent cells; development of new antigens on cell surfaces, such as the tumor specific antigens (TSA) in neoplasms produced by viruses; and the appearance of a great variety of karyotypic abnormalities in the nucleus. In vitro, neoplastic cells show decreased contact inhibition, growth on soft agar, and continuous proliferation, being potentially immortal. The loss of cell cohesiveness is associated with a decrease in calcium ion concentration and an increase of negative electric charges at the cell borders. Cell membrane alterations may be fundamental to the ability of malignant cells to escape normal control mechanisms in cell societies and invade adjacent tissues and metastasize. Most cancers arise by malignant transformation of a single cell (clonal origin); some derive from a group of altered cells (field cancerization).

The known causes of cancer include hereditary defects, ionizing radiation, chemical carcinogens, and living agents. Hereditary defects are presumably due to randomly acquired mutations. Three conditions associated with malignant tumor formation are inherited, two as dominant genes. These are some cases of retinoblastoma, familial polyposis of the colon, and xeroderma pigmentosum of the skin.

A number of neoplasms are associated with specific chromosomal defects in malignant cells. In about 90 percent of cases of chronic myelocytic leukemia, the Philadelphia chromosome, in which a portion of a chromosome 22 is translocated on number 9, is present.

Various translocations are found in some cases of acute myeloblastic and lymphoblastic leukemia and in non-Hodgkins lymphomas. In cases of retinoblastoma, there is often a deletion in the long arm of a chromosome 13, and children with birth defects associated with Wilms' tumor of the kidney have deletion in the short arm of a chromosome 11. Patients with Down's syndrome, in which there is a defect in the 21 chromosomes in body cells, have an increased incidence of acute leukemia in childhood.

Ionizing radiation causes cancer. The mechanism is not entirely clear, but it is probably an alteration in cellular DNA. A relatively high dose and a relatively long time are required for the process to take place. When these conditions exist, a wide variety of malignant tumors may arise, the kind depending especially on the tissue exposed, the intensity of the ionization, and the duration of the exposure. Ultraviolet radiation in sunlight causes skin cancer after prolonged and excessive exposure.

Numerous chemical agents cause cancer. Carcinogenic materials in coal tar include benzpyrene, methylcholanthrene, and derivatives of anthracene. The aromatic amines are known to be carcinogenic, and naphthylamines selectively cause cancer of the urinary bladder. Occupational exposure is a risk of the aniline dye industry. Vinyl chloride has been implicated in the causation of angiosarcoma of the liver. Arsenic induces papillomas and carcinomas of the skin, and asbestos causes mesothelioma of the pleura and peritoneum, as well as bronchogenic carcinoma. Agent Orange, which contains dioxin, has been implicated as a cause of Hodgkin's disease, non-Hodgkin's lymphoma, and soft tissue sarcomas.

A number of the cancer chemotherapeutic drugs, especially the alkylating agents and antibiotics, have proved to be carcinogenic. Children and immunosuppressed patients are especially susceptible to the development of a second malignant neoplasm following the use of anticancer drugs.

The mechanism of chemical carcinogenesis is not completely known. It is considered to be at least a 2-stage process. Some chemical carcinogens act as initiators, producing discrete, irreversible, additive, and transmissible dose-dependent effects on cell DNA. Other chemicals, such as croton oil, act as promoters, probably by stimulating cell division. Chemical agents most likely induce malignant transformation in cells by binding to and altering cell DNA.

Extensive epidemiologic evidence implicates diet and nutritional status in the incidence of certain forms of cancer, especially carcinoma of the breast, stomach, and colon. The exact relationship of diet and nutrition to cancer is unclear. Breast, prostate, and colon carcinoma are especially common in populations with a high fat and caloric intake. Colon carcinoma is positively related to low fiber content in the diet. Stomach carcinoma is especially common where large amounts of nitrate preservatives and small amounts of vitamin C are ingested. The vitamin C inhibits the conversion of nitrites to carcinogenic nitrosamines.

With respect to living agents, viruses have the principal role in carcinogenesis. Many oncogenic viruses have been identified in lower animals. Viruses strongly suspected as causes of human cancers are human papilloma virus (cervical carcinoma); hepatitis B virus (hepatocarcinoma); Epstein-Barr virus (Burkitt's lymphoma, nasopharyngeal carcinoma); and human T cell leukemia viruses (HTLV I and HTLV II) (T cell-hairy cell leukemia).

Oncogenes, when expressed, are involved in the transformation of normal to malignant cells. They were first detected in oncogenic RNA viruses, and have been found in chemically-induced neoplasms in animals and in human cancer cells. Oncogenes are also present in the

DNA of normal cells as potential transforming genes (proto-oncogenes). Normally they are controlled within cell DNA by regulator genes. Loss of such control and activation of an oncogene appears to be one step in the multistep process of cell transformation.

Other living agents are associated with tumor formation although a direct causal relationship is not established. Bacterial infections, especially when associated with chronic draining sinuses, may be complicated by tumor formation in the living cells of the sinus tract. Certain parasitic ova are also associated with cancer - <u>Schistosoma haematobium</u> with carcinoma of the urinary bladder, <u>S</u>. <u>mansoni</u> with cancer of the colon. Aflatoxin, a metabolic product of the fungus <u>Aspergillus flavus</u>, has been found to be a potent hepatocarcinogen.

Immune responses play an important role in the body's reaction to a malignant neoplasm. Most cancerous cells have tumor specific surface antigens. Tumors produced by a virus cross-react with others caused by the same virus. Those produced by chemical and physical agents usually have unique antigens on their cell surfaces. Both humoral and cell-mediated immune responses to tumor cells have been identified. Patients in whom a striking lymphocytic infiltration is found about and within neoplastic tissue generally have a better prognosis than those with a few stromal lymphocytes. In cases of primary immune deficiency diseases, the likelihood of development of a malignant neoplasm is ten thousand times greater than in age-matched controls. Cancer also occurs significantly more frequently in patients under immunosuppression by drugs than the expected rate. It is possible that the development of a malignant neoplasm depends on a failure of the body's immune surveillance to detect the presence of cells with foreign antigens.

Items 61-64

61. A 45 year-old man presented with hyperpigmentation of the skin, ascites, and abnormal liver function tests. His serum iron was 210 μg/dL, and the transferrin saturation was 90 percent. The most likely diagnosis is

    (A)   erythropoietic porphyria
    (B)   hepatic porphyria
    (C)   iron intoxication
    (D)   primary hemochromatosis
    (E)   secondary hemochromatosis

62. Organs which are the site of significant iron deposition in primary hemochromatosis include all of the following **EXCEPT**:

    (A)   brain
    (B)   heart
    (C)   liver
    (D)   pancreas
    (E)   skin

63. Pathologic changes or clinical manifestations which occur in patients with primary hemochromatosis include all of the following **EXCEPT**:

   (A) congestive heart failure
   (B) diabetes mellitus
   (C) hepatocarcinoma
   (D) photosensitivity dermatitis
   (E) testicular atrophy

64. Secondary hemochromatosis is most likely to occur in patients

   (A) with Addison's disease
   (B) with high dietary iron content
   (C) with malaria
   (D) with porphyria
   (E) requiring multiple blood transfusions

ANSWERS AND TUTORIAL ON ITEMS 61-64

The answers are: **61-D; 62-A; 63-D; 64-E.** Primary (endogenous) hemochromatosis is a rare disturbance of iron pigment metabolism, usually occurring in middle-aged males. It is inherited as an autosomal recessive, with incomplete expression. An association with HLA-A3 and HLA-B14 antigens has been noted. The hemochromatosis gene is on chromosome 6, tightly linked to the HLA region. There appears to be an inborn defect in the duodenal mucosa; absorption of a greatly increased amount of iron results. The total body iron may reach 50 gm. In the skin, hemosiderin deposits occur in the dermis about sweat glands, and there is also an increase in melanin deposition in the epidermis. The pancreas is usually slightly enlarged, firm, and deeply pigmented. The liver is usually enlarged, rusty red or ochre in color, and nodular. The lobules are separated by dense fibrous tissue (pigmentary cirrhosis). Hemosiderin is found mainly in the hepatic parenchymal cells. In about 7 percent of the cases of pigmentary cirrhosis, a hepatocarcinoma develops. Significant amounts of hemosiderin are deposited in the myocardial fibers and may contribute to the development of cardiac failure.

Secondary (exogenous) hemochromatosis occurs in cases of chronic refractory anemia, especially in those receiving multiple blood transfusions, and prolonged intravenous or oral iron therapy. This rare form of hemochromatosis occurs at any age and in males and females about equally. Diabetes mellitus and full-blown hepatic cirrhosis are rare. In contrast to primary hemochromatosis, in the secondary form hemosiderin pigment is deposited mainly in reticuloendothelial cells, with a lesser involvement of epithelial cells. In patients on hemodialysis for chronic renal disease, heavy iron deposits may be present in the liver and spleen even when the bone marrow is iron depleted.

65.   A 40 year-old woman has jaundice and right upper quadrant discomfort. She has not been
taking any drugs. Her serum aspartate aminotransferase is slightly elevated, bilirubin
increased (mainly direct reacting), alkaline phosphatase markedly elevated, prothrombin
time increased, and urine urobilinogen decreased. The most likely diagnosis is

   (A)   Dubin-Johnson syndrome
   (B)   Gilbert's syndrome
   (C)   hemolytic jaundice
   (D)   common duct obstruction by gallstone
   (E)   viral hepatitis

In Items 66-69, match each item with the type of jaundice typically associated with it.

      (A)   jaundice due to increased bilirubin load
      (B)   jaundice due to disturbance of bilirubin transport in hepatocytes
      (C)   jaundice due to disturbance of bilirubin conjugation in hepatocytes
      (D)   jaundice due to intrahepatic cholestasis
      (E)   jaundice due to posthepatic cholestasis

66.   carcinoma of head of the pancreas

67.   Crigler-Najjar syndrome

68.   methyltestosterone use

69.   thalassemia

In Items 70-77, match each laboratory finding with the type or types of jaundice in which it would typically be found.

(A)　jaundice due to hepatocellular necrosis
(B)　jaundice due to posthepatic obstruction
(C)　both
(D)　neither

70.　elevated serum albumin

71.　elevated serum cholesterol

72.　elevated serum bilirubin

73.　elevated serum alkaline phosphatase ($> 3X$ normal)

74.　elevated serum globulin

75.　elevated serum AST and LDH ($> 8X$ normal)

76.　increased prothrombin time

77.　decreased urine urobilinogen

ANSWERS AND TUTORIAL ON ITEMS 65-77

The answers are: **65-D; 66-E; 67-C; 68-D; 69-A; 70-D; 71-B; 72-C; 73-B; 74-A; 75-A; 76-C; 77-B**.

> Jaundice (icterus) is a condition in which there are hyperbilirubinemia and deposition of bile pigments leading to yellow, orange, or green discoloration of the skin, sclerae, and mucous membranes. Jaundice may be produced by increased bilirubin load; disturbance in bilirubin transport; disturbance of bilirubin conjugation; and disturbance of bilirubin excretion. The patient in Item 65 most likely has a disturbance in bilirubin excretion due to posthepatic duct obstruction. In middle-aged females, the commonest cause is a gallstone in the common bile duct.

Jaundice resulting from an excessive bilirubin load occurs in the hemolytic anemias and in shunt hyperbilirubinemia. In Gilbert's disease (constitutional hepatic dysfunction), the cause of the jaundice may be a defect in bilirubin transport from the serum to the site of conjugation within hepatocytes. Jaundice resulting from disturbance in bilirubin conjugation occurs in physiologic jaundice in the newborn and the Crigler-Najjar syndrome, due to a congenital deficiency or absence of glucuronyl transferase.

Disturbance of bilirubin excretion may occur within the liver or extrahepatically. Intrahepatic excretory disturbances occur in the Dubin-Johnson syndrome, cholestatic drug jaundice, viral hepatitis, and primary biliary cirrhosis. Chronic idiopathic jaundice (Dubin-Johnson syndrome) is characterized by chronic or intermittent jaundice in adolescents or young adults, with little loss of hepatic function. Cholestatic drug jaundice may be of the chlorpromazine type, which is allergic in nature, or of the testosterone type.

Jaundice may be classified as unconjugated or conjugated jaundice or prehepatic, hepatic (hepatocellular or hepatocanalicular), or posthepatic. In unconjugated jaundice, the defect in bilirubin metabolism lies in the inability of the liver cells to remove an increased, or sometimes normal, amount of bile pigment from the blood. Conjugated jaundice is due to a leakage or regurgitation of bile pigment into the bloodstream. This is caused by necrosis of hepatic cells, which swell to compress the bile canaliculi and plug them with debris, and by obstruction of the extrahepatic bile passages.

Prehepatic jaundice is actually hepatogenous. Although the etiologic hyperbilirubinemia is due to a sudden hemolysis, the jaundice results from the inability of the liver cells to remove the increased amount of circulating bilirubin. Intrahepatic (hepatogenous) jaundice may be hepatocellular and/or hepatocanalicular in origin. In the hepatocellular type, the icterus is due to a defect in hepatic cell functions of converting bilirubin to bilirubin diglucuronide and excreting the bilirubin. In the hepatocanalicular type, the cause is damage to or obstruction of the fine intrahepatic biliary passages. Most cases of hepatogenous jaundice are mixed, because in a disease process producing hepatocytic necrosis, swelling of the affected cells often obstructs the bile canaliculi and small ducts by compression.

Laboratory findings are often variable in jaundice, especially in cases due to parenchymatous hepatic damage. The decreased serum albumin in hepatogenous jaundice is due to a reduced capacity of injured hepatocytes to synthesize albumin. Elevation of serum globulin is caused by an increase in γ-globulin production in many types of liver disease. Hepatocellular necrosis releases a number of enzymes, such as aspartate aminotransferase and lactic dehydrogenase, which are then found in elevated levels in the serum. The elevated levels of serum alkaline phosphatase in both hepatogenous and posthepatic jaundice result from the regurgitation of alkaline phosphatase synthesized in the hepatocytes. Obstruction of bile outflow stimulates alkaline phosphatase synthesis in the liver. The rise in alkaline phosphatase is generally much higher in posthepatic obstruction. Decreased serum cholesterol levels in cases of hepatocellular injury results from diminished synthesis. Increased levels in posthepatic jaundice are due to increased cholesterol synthesis and regurgitation of cholesterol into the blood secondary to biliary obstruction.

While the degree of elevation of both conjugated and unconjugated serum bilirubin is quite variable in hepatogenous jaundice, the increase is typically mainly in unconjugated bilirubin. However, the conjugated bilirubin fraction may be increased more than the unconjugated form. In posthepatic jaundice the increase is principally in direct-acting bilirubin because of the regurgitation of the conjugated form into the blood secondary to the biliary obstruction.

The prothrombin time is prolonged in both hepatogenous and obstructive jaundice. In the former, the prolongation is due to decreased synthesis of prothrombin (and other coagulation factors) by the injured liver cells. The increased prothrombin time in obstructive jaundice results from decreased absorption of fat-solvent soluble vitamin K from the intestine due to the deficiency or absence of bile salts.

In hemolytic episodes severe enough to cause jaundice there is an increase in fecal and urinary urobilinogen. This occurs because there is an increased secretion of bile in hemolytic types of jaundice. In obstructive jaundice, the amount of bile reaching the intestine is decreased, so that urobilinogen and urobilin formation is lessened. The feces become light brown or even clay-colored, depending on the degree of obstruction.

Items 78-81

78.   The pigment deposited in the liver and spleen in cases of malaria and schistosomiasis is chemically closely related to

  (A)   bilirubin
  (B)   ferritin
  (C)   hematin
  (D)   hematoporphyrin
  (E)   hemosiderin

79.   All of the following are common findings in acute intermittent hepatic porphyria **EXCEPT**:

  (A)   burgundy wine colored urine
  (B)   increased urinary excretion of δ-amino levulinic acid
  (C)   large amounts of porphyrin precursors in liver
  (D)   decreased serum ceruloplasmin level
  (E)   neuropsychiatric manifestations

80.   Increased melanin pigmentation occurs in the skin in all of the following **EXCEPT**:

  (A)   Addison's disease (adrenal cortical atrophy)
  (B)   Albright's syndrome (fibrous dysplasia of bones)
  (C)   leprosy
  (D)   neurofibromatosis
  (E)   primary hemochromatosis

81.   All of the following are characteristically found in cases of ochronosis **EXCEPT**:

  (A)   alkaptonuria
  (B)   arthritis
  (C)   deposition of melanin-like pigment
  (D)   photosensitivity
  (E)   recessively transmitted inheritance

The answers are: **78-C; 79-D; 80-C; 81-D**. Hematin is an abnormal breakdown product of hemoglobin, appearing in some hemolytic crises. It rapidly combines with blood protein to form methemalbumin and appears in the tissues as brownish pigment resembling hemosiderin. It may appear in the renal tubules in massive hemoglobinuria, such as in transfusion reactions, due to the action of the acid in the urine on the hemoglobin.

Malarial pigment is closely related to hematin. Massive amounts of brown pigment are found in the reticuloendothelial cells of the liver and spleen. Schistosomal pigment is practically identical in composition and distribution.

Hematoporphyrins are iron-free pigments normally present in minute amounts in the blood and urine. They appear in higher concentrations in the porphyrias, in which there is excessive formation of uroporphyrins and coproporphyrins. The porphyrias are due to defects in porphyrin metabolism.

In acute intermittent hepatic porphyria, uroporphyrins and coproporphyrins are excreted in the urine and feces in increased amounts, along with the porphyrin precursors, porphobilinogen and δ-amino levulinic acid. This disorder occurs more often in females than males. Sunlight may precipitate neuropsychiatric signs. Burgundy wine colored urine may be excreted. Liver biopsies reveal large amounts of porphyrin precursors and variable amounts of porphyrins.

Melanin is a brownish black pigment forming the normal coloring material of the skin, iris, and elsewhere. In Addison's disease, there is bronzing of the skin due to melanin accumulation, especially in areas exposed to sunlight. Other disease states demonstrating increased melanin pigmentation include hemochromatosis (with iron pigments); multiple neurofibromatosis (café au lait spots); fibrous dysplasia of bone (Albright's syndrome); pregnancy; ACTH-producing neoplasms; tuberculosis; cachexia (patchy hyperpigmentation); urticaria pigmentosa; nevi; and melanoma.

Decreased melanin pigmentation occurs in: albinism (congenital deficiency or absence of melanin); vitiligo or leukoderma (patchy areas of depigmentation); burn or wound scars; pinta (irregular or patchy areas of depigmentation); and leprosy (due to nerve involvement).

Ochronosis in its endogenous form is a rare, recessively transmitted, congenital disorder of melanin-like pigmentation due to an inborn error in tyrosine metabolism. There is a deficiency of homogentisic acid oxidase. Homogentisic acid (an intermediate in the oxidation of tyrosine) is not oxidized, so that it accumulates in the extracellular fluid. The compound is selectively deposited in cartilage, which becomes ochre colored or black due to melanin-like pigment. Deposits within synovia produce ochronotic arthritis, and involvement of the intervertebral disks may result in an ankylosing spondylitis with development of a poker spine.

Items 82-90

In Items 82 to 89, match each item with the poison most closely related to it.

(A) carbon monoxide
(B) cyanide
(C) ethylene glycol
(D) heroin
(E) inorganic mercury
(F) lead
(G) lye
(H) methyl alcohol
(I) organic phosphates
(J) salicylates

82. acid-fast intranuclear inclusions in kidneys

83. calcium oxalate crystals in kidneys

84. blockage of cytochrome oxidase system

85. decreased O_2-carrying capacity of erythrocytes

86. decreased cholinesterase activity in erythrocytes

87. esophageal stricture

88. increased urinary coproporphyrin level

89. pulmonary edema with frothy fluid from nostrils

90. All of the following are features of fetal alcohol syndrome **EXCEPT**:

(A) abnormally low body weight
(B) hirsutism
(C) interventricular septal defect
(D) mental deficiency
(E) microphthalmos (small eyes)

ANSWERS AND TUTORIAL ON ITEMS 82-90

The answers are: **82-F; 83-C; 84-B; 85-A; 86-I; 87-G; 88-F; 89-D; 90-C.** Carbon monoxide causes decreased O_2-carrying capacity of red cells by the formation of carboxyhemoglobin, which not only displaces O_2 but interferes with the dissociation of O_2 from hemoglobin. Cyanides are potent poisons because they interfere with cellular oxidation by blocking the cytochrome oxidase system. A characteristic of ethylene glycol poisoning is the precipitation of wheat sheaf-shaped crystals of calcium oxalate in the renal tubular epithelium and lumina. Heroin overdose produces a massive pulmonary edema, often with fluid pouring from the nostrils. Lead poisoning is typified by the presence of acid-fast inclusion bodies in proximal convoluted tubular renal epithelium and increased urinary coproporphyrin levels due to interference with heme synthesis in erythroblasts. Lye, a mixture of sodium hydroxide and carbonate, is an alkaline corrosive poison which, when swallowed, causes damage to the esophageal wall which produces a stricture of the lumen by contracture of the resultant scar. Organic phosphates cause a decreased cholinesterase activity in red cells as well as at motor end plates in muscles.

The fetal alcohol syndrome occurs in infants of chronically alcoholic mothers. Common findings include prenatal and postnatal growth deficiency, small head size, mental deficiency, ocular anomalies such as microphthalmos (small eyes), cleft palate, pectus excavatum (funnel chest), and hirsutism.

Items 91-98

91.   A diabetic patient developed a carbuncle. Aspirated pus grew out <u>Staphylococcus aureus</u>. Hematogenous complications of such a staphylococcal infection include all of the following **EXCEPT**:

    (A)   endocarditis
    (B)   hepatitis
    (C)   lung abscesses
    (D)   osteomyelitis
    (E)   pyelonephritis

92.   The exotoxin produced by <u>Corynebacterium diphtheriae</u> causes pathologic changes in all of the following **EXCEPT**:

    (A)   myocardium
    (B)   pharynx
    (C)   peripheral nerves
    (D)   skeletal muscles
    (E)   trachea

93. All of the following conditions are most often due to hematogenous spread of the causative organism **EXCEPT**:

   (A)   disseminated intravascular coagulation (DIC)
   (B)   meningitis
   (C)   miliary tuberculosis
   (D)   pyelonephritis due to Escherichia coli
   (E)   typhoid fever (stage of local injury)

94. A 4 year-old child developed paroxysms of violent coughing. Whooping cough was diagnosed. The characteristic cellular reaction to infection by Bordetella pertussis is

   (A)   eosinophilic
   (B)   granulomatous
   (C)   lymphocytic
   (D)   monocytic
   (E)   neutrophilic

95. Ulcers of the ileum over enlarged Peyer's patches are a characteristic finding in

   (A)   Salmonella gastroenteritis
   (B)   Shigella dysentery
   (C)   staphylococcal gastroenteritis
   (D)   tuberculosis of the intestine
   (E)   typhoid fever

96. Of the following bacteria, the one which is **LEAST** likely to be the cause of abscess formation is

   (A)   Escherichia coli
   (B)   Proteus vulgaris
   (C)   Pseudomonas aeruginosa
   (D)   Salmonella typhi
   (E)   Staphylococcus aureus

97. The typical cell of reaction in typhoid fever is the

   (A)   eosinophil
   (B)   lymphocyte
   (C)   macrophage
   (D)   neutrophil
   (E)   plasma cell

98.   Infarct-like foci secondary to an acute suppurative arteritis are found in infections due to

    (A)   Clostridium perfringens
    (B)   Escherichia coli
    (C)   Proteus vulgaris
    (D)   Pseudomonas aeruginosa
    (E)   Yersinia pestis

ANSWERS AND TUTORIAL ON ITEMS 91-98

The answers are: **91-B; 92-D; 93-D; 94-C; 95-E; 96-D; 97-C; 98-D**.

> Hematogenous spread with septicemia and localization of Staphylococcus aureus is common. Heart valves, meninges, bone, and kidneys are often sites of hematogenous infection by S. aureus and other bacteria. However, E. coli pyelonephritis is usually due to an ascending infection from the lower urinary tract. Lung abscesses may be due to bacteremia or septic embolism, although they are most often due to inhaled organisms. Blood stream dissemination of gram-negative bacteria may produce DIC by release of their endotoxins. Salmonella typhi bacteremia results in local lesions in the ileum, lymph nodes, and spleen. Miliary granulomata in many sites are caused by blood stream spread of M. tuberculosis.

Items 99-106

In Items 99-103, match the changes with the type or types of tuberculosis with which each is typically associated.

      (A)   primary infection tuberculosis
      (B)   reinfection tuberculosis
      (C)   both
      (D)   neither

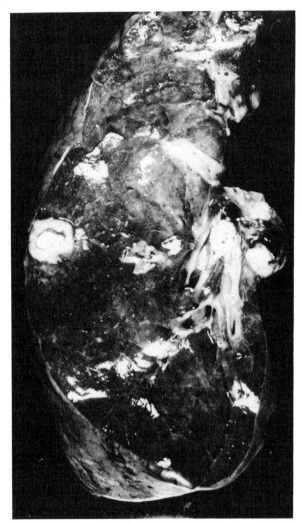

99.   apical lesion in the lung

100.   cavity formation in the lung

101.   lesions in Figure 1.8 at right

102.   hilar lymph node involvement

103.   positive tuberculin skin test

Figure 1.8

104. The finding of caseating granulomas in a tissue section is specifically diagnostic of

    (A)   histoplasmosis
    (B)   leprosy
    (C)   sarcoidosis
    (D)   tuberculosis
    (E)   none of the above

105. A 25 year-old man developed cervical lymphadenopathy. On chest X-ray the hilar nodes were enlarged, and there were pulmonary infiltrates. A tentative diagnosis of sarcoidosis was made. All of the following statements are correct concerning sarcoidosis **EXCEPT**:

    (A)   the cause is unknown
    (B)   noncaseating granulomas in lesions are diagnostic
    (C)   asteroid bodies may be found in giant cells
    (D)   the eyes and parotid glands may be involved (uveoparotid fever)
    (E)   the lungs and lymph nodes are the most commonly involved sites

106. A 30 year-old woman using an intrauterine device developed pelvic inflammatory disease. The likeliest causative organism is

    (A)   Actinomyces israelii
    (B)   Candida albicans
    (C)   Chlamydia trachomatis
    (D)   Nocardia asteroides
    (E)   Trichomonas vaginalis

ANSWERS AND TUTORIAL ON ITEMS 99-106

The answers are: **99-B; 100-B; 101-A; 102-A; 103-C; 104-E; 105-B; 106-A.**

In Item 101, Figure 1.8 shows a Ghon complex, which is characteristic of primary tuberculosis. In reference to Item 104, the specific diagnosis of a case with caseating granulomas depends on identifying the causative organism on smear or culture. In Item 105, sarcoidosis is a diagnosis of exclusion in which all other known causes of noncaseating granulomas have been ruled out.

Tuberculosis is a specific infectious granulomatous disease due to Mycobacterium tuberculosis. The human strain is the chief cause of tuberculosis of all organ systems at all ages in man. The bovine strain may cause human tuberculosis, especially of the tonsils, cervical lymph nodes, and gastrointestinal tract in children. Numerous cases are due to atypical mycobacteria, such as M. kansasii and avium intracellulare. The latter is especially associated with AIDS patients.

An important source of human infection is direct contact with persons having open tuberculous lung lesions, i.e., tuberculous cavities communicating with bronchi. These cavities contain great numbers of living organisms. This type of exposure gives rise to exogenous infection. Also important is endogenous infection, meaning reinfection of an individual as a result of the breakdown of his or her own old tuberculous lesions. The chief portal of entry of the organism is the respiratory tract. Bacilli may be inhaled directly by droplet infection or indirectly in contaminated dust. Pulmonary tuberculosis is the result of entry of organisms by this avenue.

First infection (primary) tuberculosis is the usual form of tuberculosis in children and young adults. The parenchymal lung lesion (Ghon lesion) is usually subpleural in the periphery of the lower lobe of one lung. The parenchymal lung lesion plus the lesions in the regional lymph nodes are known as the primary (Ghon) complex. Reinfection tuberculosis is the usual form of tuberculosis in adults. It features parenchymal lung lesions with no lymph node lesions. Cavities are common, usually in the apices of the upper lobes of the lungs.

In progressive tuberculosis, tubercle bacilli may be disseminated within the host by: direct extension, involving contiguous tissues; natural passages, such as along the bronchial tree from an upper lobe cavity to a lower lobe on the same or opposite side; lymphatic channels to regional lymph nodes (this method is practically restricted to first-infection tuberculosis); hematogenous spread, resulting in miliary tuberculosis; or implantation in a body cavity.

Miliary tuberculosis is the consequence of tuberculous bacteremia, either via the thoracic duct and the superior vena cava in first-infection tuberculosis, or more rarely by dissemination of bacilli from an eroded vein in reinfection tuberculosis. Small (1 to 2 mm.) caseous lesions appear in the lungs, liver, spleen, meninges, kidneys, and in almost any other organ. Cold abscesses signify liquefied tuberculous lesions similar to pyogenic abscesses but lacking the clinical features of acute inflammation. The liquefied material burrows along fascial planes in the direction of least resistance. Such a lesion beginning in a thoracic vertebra may extend along the sheath of the psoas muscle to a point in the groin (psoas abscess). If it ruptures through the skin, a tuberculous sinus forms and may persist for months or years.

Sarcoidosis is a chronic granulomatous disease that is characterized pathologically by noncaseating granulomas and chemically by an increase in serum globulin. Early lesions are about the size of miliary tubercles. They are composed of great numbers of epithelioid cells, with a ring of lymphocytes in some instances, and often with giant cells that resemble Langhans' cells. The giant cells sometimes contain crystalline material, asteroid bodies, or laminated iron-containing structures (Schaumann bodies). The calcified star-shaped asteroid bodies consist of a core of collagen fibers. The Schaumann body results from the deposition of iron and calcium salts on mucopolysaccharides. Sarcoid granulomas may occur in almost any organ or tissue. They are most common in the lungs (about 90 percent of cases), lymph nodes (90 percent), and liver and spleen (75 percent). The myocardium is involved in about 20 percent.

The cause of actinomycosis is Actinomyces israelii, a higher bacterium, especially in farmers. Infections of the jaw (lumpy jaw) arise through breaks in the buccal mucosa from chewing grain or through the root of a carious tooth. Primary lesions of the intestines are due to ingestion and of the lungs, to inhalation. The most common lesion occurs in the lower jaw and neck. A firm mass develops, breaks down, and becomes riddled with abscesses, multiple sinuses opening onto the skin. Microscopically, the lesions are granulomatous (fibrosis, lymphocytes, epithelioid cells, and multinucleated giant cells) and suppurative (clusters of neutrophils), and contain tiny yellow sulfur granules. These granules show a central felted mass of mycelial filaments, with peripheral club-shaped bodies. <u>A. israelii</u> is a cause of pelvic inflammatory disease in women using intrauterine devices.

Items 107-114

In Items 107-111, match the changes with the stage or stages of acquired syphilis with which each is typically associated.

(A) primary syphilis
(B) secondary syphilis
(C) both
(D) neither

107. chancre

108. gumma

109. meningitis

110. mucous patch

111. presence of <u>Treponema pallidum</u> in lesions

112. Skin lesions in secondary syphilis include all of the following **EXCEPT**:

(A) condylomata lata
(B) macules
(C) papules
(D) pustules
(E) vesicles

113. A young women with secondary lesions gave birth to a child with congenital syphilis. All of the following are stigmata of congenital syphilis **EXCEPT**:

(A) a chancre
(B) Hutchinson's teeth (notched incisors)
(C) interstitial keratitis
(D) saddle nose
(E) saber shins

114. A middle-aged woman enjoyed working in her garden adjacent to the woods. She developed a slowly spreading reddish lesion on her left arm. It faded, but weeks later her knees became hot, swollen, and painful. The likeliest diagnosis is

   (A)   erysipelas
   (B)   leptospirosis (Weil's disease)
   (C)   Lyme disease
   (D)   spotted fever
   (E)   tularemia

ANSWERS AND TUTORIAL ON ITEMS 107-114

The answers are: **107-A; 108-D; 109-D; 110-B; 111-C; 112-E; 113-A; 114-C**. Syphilis is due to <u>Treponema</u> <u>pallidum.</u> The only known source of infection in syphilis is another infected human being. Since the organisms die rapidly on exposure to air, direct contact with syphilitic lesions is necessary for transmission of the disease. In about 95 percent of the cases, this contact is venereal, by direct inoculation of the genitalia with living organisms from an open lesion on the genitals of a sexual partner. The fetus in utero may be infected from a syphilitic placenta, which in turn is infected from a syphilitic mother.

   The chancre is the lesion characteristic of the primary stage of syphilis, and appears 2 to 6 weeks after infection. It occurs at the site of inoculation; it is usually seen on the genitals but may appear on the lips or buccal mucosa. The chancre is a firm, round, relatively painless, button-like lesion. It usually is single and generally is 0.5 to 2.0 cm in diameter. Initially papular, it later becomes superficially ulcerated. Microscopically, there is dilatation of the capillaries, and the perivascular spaces are packed with an infiltrate composed chiefly of lymphocytes, plasma cells, and macrophages. The chancre usually persists for 3 to 8 weeks and heals with little scarring.

   The characteristic lesions of the secondary stage affect chiefly the skin and mucous membranes. The interval between the disappearance of the chancre and the appearance of the skin lesions is usually 2 to 6 months. The skin lesions are macular, papular, or pustular. Alopecia (patchy hair loss) is a common feature of this stage. The most characteristic lesions of the mucous membranes in this stage are the mucous patches. These are superficial ulcers noted in the buccal mucosa and pharynx. Another mucocutaneous lesion of the secondary stage is the condyloma latum, a flat nodular lesion which occurs most often in the moist areas such as those about the anus or genitals. Microscopic examination of the skin and mucosal lesions shows numerous blood and lymphatic channels surrounded by cellular infiltrate composed chiefly of plasma cells and lymphocytes.

   After a variable interval, which may occasionally be as short as 6 months after the primary infection but is more often a matter of some years, the lesions characteristic of the tertiary stage appear. There are two general types of tertiary lesion: (1) the gumma, and (2) a diffuse inflammatory fibrosis. The gumma is a rubbery, well-defined, infarct-like lesion, usually several centimeters in diameter, occurring especially in the liver but occasionally in the testes or central nervous system. Microscopically, the outline of organ architecture can still be recognized in the necrotic zone. At the periphery of the gumma there is fibrous tissue proliferation, perivascular plasma cell and lymphocytic infiltration, and occasionally a few giant cells. In inflammatory fibrosis, there is replacement of specialized cells by fibrous connective tissue, lymphocytes, and plasma cells. The aorta and central nervous system are the sites chiefly affected.

In congenital syphilis the treponema is transmitted to the placenta and thence to the fetus. If pregnancy occurs during the primary or secondary stage of syphilis, and if the infection is untreated, the spirochetemia is usually so heavy that it causes the death of the fetus in utero and the result is a prematurely born dead child (stillbirth). A subsequent pregnancy in the same mother may result in a living child born at term but with clinical evidence of congenital syphilis.

Congenital syphilis differs from syphilis acquired in later life in several regards. There is no chancre. The syphilitic infection interferes with bone growth and results in stunting and frequently in bone deformities. Among the most characteristic syphilitic deformities are those of the nasal septum resulting in the saddle-nose, and the anterior bowing of the tibiae which gives them an unduly sharp anterior edge known as saber shin. As in syphilis of adults, the treponema produces a diffuse fibrosis of many organs, but the liver shows the most evident damage in most cases. If the infant survives the neonatal period, manifestations of syphilis may appear later, particularly skeletal deformity, defective dentition (Hutchinson's teeth), interstitial keratitis, nerve deafness, or central nervous system disease.

Lyme disease is caused by the spirochete <u>Borrelia burgdorferi</u>, transmitted by nymphs and ticks of the Ixodes genus. A few days to 3 weeks after the inoculating bite a slowly spreading red lesion appears on the skin (erythema migrans). This gradually fades. Weeks or months later some patients develop myocarditis, pericarditis, meningo-encephalitis, and/or arthritis. Synovial biopsies show an infiltration of lymphocytes and plasma cells, resembling rheumatoid arthritis. Knee and other large extremity joints become hot, swollen, and painful. This secondary phase usually clears after several months, leaving some patients with joint deformities. Tertiary cardio-vascular and neurologic signs sometimes appear, and stillbirths have been attributed to intrauterine infection.

Items 115-125

115. Following a camping trip a young man developed a hemorrhagic rash, diagnosed as spotted fever. In spotted fever, the rickettsiae are found within

    (A)   endothelial cells
    (B)   epidermal basal cells
    (C)   Kupffer cells
    (D)   macrophages
    (E)   splenic phagocytes

116. A 6 year-old child developed fever, photophobia, and malaise. A maculopapular rash appeared. The diagnosis of measles (rubeola) was made. All of the following statements about measles are true **EXCEPT**:

(A) a Koplik spot on the buccal mucosa appears early
(B) multinucleated giant cells are found in tonsils and lymph nodes
(C) epithelial giant cells are found in sputum
(D) recurrences are common due to recrudescence of the virus
(E) subacute sclerosing panencephalitis may develop years later

117. A 25 year-old woman in her first trimester of pregnancy developed rubella. Congenital anomalies caused by the rubella virus include all of the following **EXCEPT**:

(A) deafmutism
(B) interventricular septal defect
(C) lenticular cataracts
(D) persistent ductus arteriosus
(E) polycystic kidneys

118. In mumps, lesions occur in all of the following **EXCEPT**:

(A) liver
(B) meninges
(C) pancreas
(D) parotid glands
(E) testes

119. A 19 year-old college student complained of sore throat, fever, and cervical lymphadenopathy. She was diagnosed as having infectious mononucleosis. Findings include all of the following **EXCEPT**:

(A) atypical lymphocytes (Downey cells)
(B) heterophil antibody in serum
(C) leukocytosis
(D) splenomegaly
(E) vesicles on the lips (fever blisters)

120. In acquired immunodeficiency syndrome (AIDS) the immune defect is due to a

(A) depletion of CD4-helper T lymphocytes
(B) depletion of CD8-cytotoxic T lymphocytes
(C) failure of B lymphocytes to mature to plasma cells
(D) failure of pre-B lymphocytes to mature
(E) lymphoid stem cell defect

121. Opportunistic organisms which commonly infect patients with AIDS include all of the following **EXCEPT**:

    (A) Cryptosporidium
    (B) cytomegalovirus
    (C) Mycobacterium avium-intracellulare
    (D) Plasmodium ovale
    (E) Pneumocystis carinii

122. Malignant neoplasms which occur in increased incidence in patients with AIDS include all of the following **EXCEPT**:

    (A) Burkitt's lymphoma
    (B) hairy cell leukemia
    (C) immunoblastic lymphoma
    (D) Kaposi's sarcoma
    (E) primary CNS lymphoma

123. A 30 year-old diabetic with sinusitis showed signs of pulmonary consolidation. Despite treatment he developed meningitis and died. At autopsy the lungs showed thrombi in small pulmonary arteries and foci of infarction. A fungus was identified. The likeliest causative organism is

    (A) Aspergillus fumigatus
    (B) Candida albicans
    (C) Cryptococcus neoformans
    (D) Histoplasma capsulatum
    (E) Mucor corymbifer

124. On his return from a trip to South America, a 30 year-old man complained of diarrhea as well as tenesmus. Entamoeba histolytica was found in his feces. A common complication of amebic dysentery is

    (A) adrenal cortical necrosis
    (B) carrier state due to amebic cholecystitis
    (C) liver abscess
    (D) perforation of amebic ulcer in colon
    (E) sigmoid colon obstruction due to fibrosis

125.   A 60 year-old resident of northern Minnesota who was an inveterate fisherman in nearby lakes became pale and easily fatigued. He was found to have a megaloblastic anemia due to vitamin B_{12} deficiency. Further studies discovered a helminthic infestation. The causative organism is

(A)   <u>Diphyllobothrium</u> <u>latum</u>
(B)   <u>Echinococcus</u> <u>granulosus</u>
(C)   <u>Hymenolopis</u> <u>nana</u>
(D)   <u>Taenia</u> <u>saginata</u>
(E)   <u>Taenia</u> <u>solium</u>

ANSWERS AND TUTORIAL ON ITEMS 115-125

The answers are: **115-A; 116-D; 117-E; 118-A; 119-E; 120-A; 121-D; 122-B; 123-E; 124-C; 125-A**. Spotted fever is caused by <u>Rickettsia</u> <u>rickettsii</u>. Rickettsiae are gram-negative, bacterium-like, obligate intracellular parasites. Most are transmitted by ticks or mites. The gross changes are not distinctive and consist mainly of petechiae or ecchymoses. The typical microscopic change in rickettsial infections is a mononuclear cell inflammatory reaction (lymphocytes, plasmacytes, and macrophages) about small blood vessels. The rickettsiae enter the bloodstream via the bites and are carried to the capillary beds throughout the body. They enter and proliferate in the endothelial cells lining arterioles, venules, and capillaries in many parts of the body.

The gross and microscopic changes in spotted fever occur in the skin and viscera. The rickettsiae are found in the endothelial and smooth muscle cells of small blood vessels. In the brain, there are proliferation of glial tissue to form nodules, sometimes around small blood vessels; perivascular infiltration of lymphocytes, with endothelial swelling; and necrosis and thrombosis of arterioles, with small infarcts of the brain.

Rubella (German measles) is caused by a togavirus of the Rubivirus genus. Transmission is by direct contact, droplet infection, and transplacentally. Rubella is a mild childhood exanthem, the rash being maculopapular and purplish red. Numerous congenital anomalies are related to the incidence of rubella in women during the first trimester of pregnancy. Rubella virus has been isolated from defective newborns. The most common anomalies are those of the heart, deaf-mutism, microcephaly, and lenticular cataracts. The pathologic changes in childhood rubella are little known. There is a lymphocytic dermal infiltrate in the skin macules and papules.

Rubeola (measles) is caused by a paramyxovirus. Transmission of the virus is by direct contact and droplet infection from secretion of the nose, mouth, and eyes. The earliest characteristic sign is the Koplik spot a small, grayish yellow focus with a red halo on the buccal mucosa opposite the first molar. Microscopically, there is an infiltration of polymorphonuclear leukocytes, with capillary dilatation and small hemorrhages. In the skin, lesions the dermis is edematous and infiltrated by lymphocytes and macrophages. Small hemorrhages may occur. The formation of multinucleated giant cells is the most specific change in rubeola. Reticuloendothelial (Warthin-Finkeldey) giant cells, with up to 100 closely packed nuclei, are found in the tonsils, lymph nodes, spleen, and lymphatic tissue of the intestines and appendix. Epithelial giant cells have been found in the tracheobronchial mucosa and in nasal and bronchial secretions. Subacute sclerosing panencephalitis develops rarely years after clinical rubeola as a slow virus infection.

Mumps is caused by a paramyxovirus. Transmission is by droplet infection and direct contact. In about 70 percent of the cases, there is bilateral parotid involvement. Mumps is a systemic disease with localization in the parotid glands, testes or ovaries, pancreas, and meninges. The parotid glands are enlarged and pink, the edematous interstitial tissue being infiltrated by mononuclear cells. Similar changes are found in the testes. The orchitis is usually unilateral and patchy and is rarely followed by sterility. In acute meningoencephalitis, the meninges are infiltrated by lymphocytes. The brain is edematous and shows perivascular lymphocytic cuffing.

Infectious mononucleosis is a mildly contagious disease affecting adolescents and young adults. It is caused by the Epstein-Barr (EB) virus. The WBCs usually number 10,000 to 20,000/mm^3. Many immature large lymphocytes with foamy basophilic cytoplasm and indented nuclei (Downey cells) are noted in the blood smear; similar cells are also seen in the sinuses of the lymph nodes. In up to 90 percent of cases of mononucleosis, a heterophil antibody appears in the serum, capable of agglutinating sheep's red blood cells. The disease is usually mild, terminating spontaneously after a few weeks, but in some instances it is quite severe, even fatal. Hepatitis is an important complication. Massive intraperitoneal hemorrhage due to spontaneous rupture of the spleen has occurred occasionally.

Acquired immunodeficiency syndrome (AIDS) occurs in male homosexuals, drug addicts, and boys with hemophilia (due to transmission via blood products). It also develops in female sexual partners and children of patients in high risk groups. The cause of AIDS is a retrovirus, HIV1. Patients, after a usually prolonged latent period, become immunodeficient due to infection of CD4-helper T lymphocytes. This leads to their depletion, making patients susceptible to opportunistic infections and the development of cancers. Opportunistic infections include pneumonitis due to Pneumocystis carinii (often in association with the cytomegalovirus), ulcerative perianal Herpes simplex infections, atypical tuberculosis due to Mycobacterium avium-intracellulare, oral and esophageal candidiasis, cryptococcal infections, toxoplasmosis, and profuse diarrhea due to the intestinal protozoan, Cryptosporidium. Malignancies in AIDS patients include Kaposi's sarcoma (a usually rare form of blood vessel cancer) and Burkitt's, immunoblastic, and primary central nervous system lymphomas.

Amebiasis is caused by Entamoeba histolytica, a protozoan found in feces as trophozites, precystic forms, and cysts. The trophozoite, the only form found in tissues, moves by pseudopodia. Its cytoplasm may contain erythrocytes and vacuoles. Usually transmission occurs by ingestion of food or water contaminated with human feces containing cysts of E. histolytica. Food is contaminated by flies and soiled fingers of food handlers. Amebic dysentery is characterized by the formation of deep, ragged ulcers with undermined edges in the colon and rectum. Because of the undermining, amebic lesions are called flask-shaped or water-bottle ulcers. Microscopically, the margins and floor show little inflammatory reaction, with only a few macrophages and lymphocytes. Hordes of amebae are found in the submucosa. Complications of amebic dysentery include liver abscess. This is common due to infiltration of the portal venules. The abscesses are due to liquefactive necrosis of the liver cells by the proteolytic enzymes of the amebae. The wall consists of necrotic liver cells infiltrated with lymphocytes and plasma cells.

Diphyllobothrium latum (fish tapeworm) infestation is common in the northern US. There is usually a single worm, which grows to be 10 meters long. Larvae are ingested in raw fish. In about 1 percent of cases, the tapeworm ingests large enough amounts of vitamin B_{12} to cause a megaloblastic anemia in the host.

Items 126-137

126.   A 3 year-old African child had been weaned a few months before and fed with adequate amounts of carbohydrates. He failed to grow and became edematous. His hair became red, and there were flaky areas of depigmentation and hyperpigmentation of the skin. The liver was enlarged. The likeliest diagnosis is

    (A)   helminthic infestation
    (B)   kwashiorkor
    (C)   marasmus
    (D)   malabsorption syndrome
    (E)   multivitamin deficiencies

127.   The underlying cause of kwashiorkor is a

    (A)   high carbohydrate diet
    (B)   low calorie diet
    (C)   low fat diet
    (D)   low protein diet
    (E)   multiple vitamin deficiencies

128.   A 6 year-old child in southern Sudan received almost no food for weeks except for some meat from small animals his father caught. He lost weight steadily, and his arms and legs became like sticks. There was no edema or hepatomegaly. The likeliest diagnosis is

    (A)   helminthic infestation
    (B)   kwashiorkor
    (C)   marasmus
    (D)   malabsorption syndrome
    (E)   multivitamin deficiencies

129.	The underlying cause of marasmus is

(A)	low calorie diet
(B)	low carbohydrate diet
(C)	low fat diet
(D)	low protein diet
(E)	multiple vitamin deficiencies

In Items 130-135, match the change with the vitamin deficiency with which it is most closely related.

(A)	avitaminosis A
(B)	avitaminosis C
(C)	avitaminosis D
(D)	avitaminosis K
(E)	cyanocobalamin deficiency
(F)	riboflavin deficiency
(G)	niacin deficiency
(H)	thiamine deficiency

130.	hemorrhages from prothrombin deficiency

131.	night blindness (nyctalopia)

132.	erythema and hyperpigmentation of skin

133.	bone softening due to formation of osteoid that fails to calcify

134.	delayed callus formation because of deficient cartilage and osteoid formation

135.	dilated cardiomyopathy

136.	A 16 year-old girl took 100,000 units of vitamin A daily for months as a treatment for acne. All of the following occur in chronic hypervitaminosis A **EXCEPT**:

(A)	desquamation and hyperpigmentation of skin
(B)	hepatic fibrosis with Ito cells (lipid-laden Kupffer cells)
(C)	premature ossification of epiphyses
(D)	pseudotumor cerebri with papilledema
(E)	renal calculi

137. A 50 year-old man ingested large numbers of multivitamin tablets daily "to improve his health". He developed dyspnea. A chest X-ray film showed a lacy pattern of radiodensities throughout both lungs indicating metastatic calcification. His serum calcium was 14 mg/dL, phosphorus 2 mg/dL. Of the following the most likely cause is

    (A)   hypervitaminosis A
    (B)   hypervitaminosis C
    (C)   hypervitaminosis D
    (D)   hypervitaminosis K
    (E)   niacin intoxication

ANSWERS AND TUTORIAL ON ITEMS 126-137

The answers are: **126-B; 127-D; 128-C; 129-A; 130-D; 131-A; 132-G; 133-C; 134-B; 135-H; 136-E; 137-C**.

In Item 126 the history of being weaned from breast milk, edema, red hair, skin changes, and hepatomegaly are characteristic of kwashiorkor, which is due to a low protein diet. In Item 128 the starving child shows marasmus due to a low calorie diet. Of course, both kwashiorkor and marasmus often occur in the same child (marasmic kwashiorkor).

In Items 130 to 135 vitamin K is essential for synthesis of prothrombin in the liver; vitamin A is necessary for the synthesis of rhodopsin (a light sensitive pigment in the retina); niacin prevents the development of pellagra with its rough skin, diarrhea, and mental changes; vitamin D prevents rickets in children by its effect on calcification of osteoid in bones; vitamin C is essential for the development of intercellular substances including cartilaginous and bone matrix; thiamine prevents beriberi heart disease in which there is cardiac enlargement, due to dilatation, and heart failure.

Overuse of vitamins can be toxic. Hypervitaminosis A may even mimic a brain tumor by causing increased intracranial pressure. It does not produce renal stones, which do occur in hypervitaminosis D, where there is hypercalcemia (due to enhanced calcium absorption) and metastatic calcification in the lungs, kidneys, and gastric mucosa.

CHAPTER II

CARDIOVASCULAR PATHOLOGY

Items 138-141

138. The known causes of congenital cardiovascular defects include all of the following **EXCEPT**:

    (A) advanced maternal age
    (B) maternal rubella in first trimester
    (C) trisomy 13
    (D) trisomy 18
    (E) trisomy 21

139. All of the following are findings in the tetralogy of Fallot **EXCEPT**:

    (A) dextrorotation of the aorta
    (B) hypertrophy of the right ventricle
    (C) interventricular septal defect
    (D) persistent ductus arteriosus
    (E) pulmonary valvular stenosis

140. A 20 year-old woman was found to have an elevated blood pressure as measured in both arms, but the pressure in her legs was low. The most likely diagnosis is

    (A) coarctation of the aorta
    (B) Cushing's syndrome
    (C) increased intracranial pressure
    (D) pheochromocytoma
    (E) toxemia of pregnancy

141. A 20 year-old man complained of progressive difficulty in swallowing food. His problem was found to be due to a congenital cardiovascular anomaly. The defect is

    (A) aneurysm of aortic root due to Marfan's syndrome
    (B) coarctation of the aorta
    (C) patent ductus arteriosus
    (D) persistent right aortic arch
    (E) persistent truncus arteriosus

ANSWERS AND TUTORIAL ON ITEMS 138-141

The answers are: **138-A; 139-D; 140-A; 141-D**. The cause of about 90 percent of congenital cardiovascular defects are multifactorial, 5 percent are related to chromosomal disorders (Down's syndrome, trisomy 13 and 18); and 2 percent to maternal infection (rubella). The overall incidence of significant congenital cardiovascular anomalies is about 6 per 1000 births. There is approximately a threefold increase in congenital heart disease among siblings of an afflicted child. In Marfan's disease, aortic aneurysms may occur as a result of the connective tissue defect. In trisomy 21 (Down's syndrome), cardiovascular anomalies occur in about 40 percent of the cases. Almost all infants with trisomy 13 or 18 have cardiovascular malformations, especially interventricular septal defect and patent ductus arteriosus.

Cases of congenital heart disease are associated with maternal rubella during the first 8 weeks of pregnancy. In infants with the congenital rubella syndrome, about 50 percent show evidence of congenital heart disease, chiefly persistent ductus arteriosus but also interventricular septal defect.

Atrial septal defects occur about twice as often in females as in males. An ostium primum defect is caused by a failure of closure of the ostium by the septum secundum growing upward from the atrioventricular cushion. The defect is low on the interatrial septum and may involve the two atrioventricular valve rings, converting them into a single ring. Usually much less significant is the ostium secundum defect (persistent foramen ovale). Apparently due to a failure in proper development of the septum secundum, this defect is high above the valve rings and is often functionally closed by an endocardial flap, even when anatomically patent.

Interventricular septal defect (Roger's disease) is the most common congenital cardiac malformation, and may occur alone or as a part of a combined lesion such as the tetralogy of Fallot. The defect commonly occurs in the membranous portion of the septum just below the aortic valve and is usually small. Common atrioventricular canal is most often associated with Down's syndrome.

With interatrial and, more particularly, interventricular septal defects there is usually some degree of left-to-right shunt after birth, increasing pulmonary blood flow and pulmonary arterial pressure. Ordinarily there is no cyanosis. A left-to-right shunt may lead to pulmonary overload, small pulmonary vascular narrowing (obstructive pulmonary vascular disease), pulmonary hypertension, and cor pulmonale. With reversal of the shunt to right-to-left, cyanosis develops.

The most common of the major combined cardiac lesions is the tetralogy of Fallot. Of the four defects, the most significant is the narrowing of the out-flow tract from the right ventricle (pulmonic stenosis). This results in high pressure, causing right ventricular hypertrophy and preventing closure of the interventricular septal defect. The fourth defect is dextroposition of the aorta, which arises over the septum, receiving blood from both left and right ventricles. Cyanosis is usually present from birth ("blue baby") due to inadequate oxygenation of the blood as a result of diminished pulmonary blood flow.

Transposition of the aorta and pulmonary artery, i.e., the aorta arising from the right ventricle and the pulmonary artery arising from the left ventricle, is a most serious congenital anomaly. It occurs in boys 4 times as often as in girls. Cyanosis is usually present at birth. Mortality is 85 percent in the first 6 months of life. Survival is possible only when a septal defect or patent ductus arteriosus is present. An interventricular septal defect is present in about 1/3 of cases. In "corrected" transposition, the ventricles are also reversed so that the venous ventricle gives rise to the pulmonary artery and the arterial ventricle, to the aorta. The atrioventricular valves are reversed, the tricuspid valve being in the left ventricle and the bicuspid in the right one.

Persistence of the ductus arteriosus after birth often results from an intrinsic abnormality in the ductus itself. Rubella infection in early pregnancy is commonly associated with patent ductus. Blood is usually shunted from the aorta to the pulmonary artery, resulting in a low diastolic pressure in the systemic circulation and a wide pulse pressure. The increased pulmonary blood flow gradually causes pulmonary hypertension, resulting eventually in reversal of the shunt; cyanosis usually becomes evident at this time. Patent ductus is found in girls about 3 times as often as in boys.

Coarctation of the aorta may occur at either of two sites: just proximal to the ligamentum arteriosum, in which case it is known as the infantile type, or just distal to the ligamentum, known as the adult type. The former is usually associated with persistence of the ductus while the latter is often associated with a great increase in the collateral arterial circulation of the thorax. Regardless of its site, the effect of coarctation is diminished blood flow below the constriction. The blood pressure in the arms is elevated while that in the legs is lower than normal. Coarctation occurs about 4 times as often in boys as in girls. Bicuspid aortic valve is often associated with the adult type.

Persistent right aortic arch ordinarily causes no difficulty, but the ligamentum arteriosum may pass behind the trachea and esophagus forming a vascular ring which compresses these structures, causing difficulty in swallowing, which may not become apparent until adulthood.

Items 142-158

A 10 year-old child had a ß-hemolytic streptococcal pharyngitis from which she recovered on penicillin therapy. A month later she became ill again with fever, joint swelling, involuntary movements, and a skin rash. The diagnosis of acute rheumatic fever was made.

142.   All of the following laboratory finds are typically present during an attack of acute rheumatic fever **EXCEPT**:

   (A)   elevated antistreptolysin titer
   (B)   elevated erythrocyte sedimentation rate
   (C)   increased C-reactive protein level
   (D)   leukocytosis
   (E)   positive throat culture for ß-hemolytic streptococci

143. Typical lesions in acute rheumatic fever include all of the following **EXCEPT**:

   (A) erythema marginatum
   (B) polyarthritis
   (C) poststreptococcal glomerulonephritis
   (D) subcutaneous nodules
   (E) verrucae on mitral valve

144. The most characteristic lesion in acute rheumatic myocarditis is the Aschoff body. Microscopic features of the Aschoff body include all of the following **EXCEPT**:

   (A) eosinophils
   (B) fibrinoid necrosis
   (C) lymphocytes
   (D) multinucleated (Aschoff) cells
   (E) perivascular location

145. A 30 year-old woman, who had scarlet fever when she was 10, was found to have a cardiac murmur. She was diagnosed as having rheumatic heart disease. The type of valvular lesion most closely related to this disease is

   (A) aortic insufficiency
   (B) aortic stenosis
   (C) mitral stenosis
   (D) pulmonic stenosis
   (E) tricuspid stenosis

146. A 25 year-old woman was found to have a midsystolic click and was diagnosed as having floppy valve syndrome. The cause of the floppy valve is

   (A) chronic rheumatic valvulitis
   (B) fenestration of a valve leaflet
   (C) increased circumference of the mitral annulus
   (D) myxomatous degeneration of valve leaflets
   (E) rupture of a papillary muscle

147. Floppy valve syndrome most commonly involves the

   (A) aortic valve
   (B) mitral valve
   (C) mitral and aortic valves
   (D) pulmonic valve
   (E) tricuspid valve

148. A 60 year-old man collapsed while playing golf. He was found to have heart block and an aortic systolic murmur transmitted into the neck. The most likely cause is

   (A)   bicuspid aortic valve
   (B)   calcific aortic stenosis
   (C)   fungal endocarditis with coronary embolism
   (D)   hypertrophic subaortic stenosis
   (E)   syphilitic involvement of aortic valve

In Items 149-158, match the items with the form or forms of bacterial endocarditis with which each is most closely related.

   (A)   acute bacterial endocarditis
   (B)   subacute bacterial endocarditis
   (C)   both
   (D)   neither

149. α-hemolytic streptococci (S. viridans)

150. bacteremia

151. development on normal valves

152. disseminated lupus erythematosus

153. focal glomerulonephritis

154. perforation of valve cusps

155. Roth's spots (retinal hemorrhages)

156. septic embolism

157. terminal (marantic) endocarditis

158. valvular prostheses

The answers are: **142-E; 143-C; 144-A; 145-C; 146-D; 147-B; 148-B; 149-B; 150-C; 151-A; 152-D; 153-B; 154-A; 155-B; 156-A; 157-D; 158-A**.

Weeks before the development of rheumatic fever the related streptococcal infection has cleared, so there would be no positive throat culture. Poststreptococcal glomerulonephritis does not develop concomitantly with rheumatic fever often, although they share a remote causative factor. While the Aschoff body is due to an immunologic reaction, there are no eosinophils in it. Both rheumatic heart disease and floppy valve syndrome most often affect the mitral valve. Myxomatous degeneration is responsible for the floppiness of the floppy valve. Calcific aortic stenosis is characterized by an aortic systolic murmur and heart block due to compression of the conduction bundle.

α-hemolytic streptococci cause the less virulent subacute bacterial endocarditis (SBE), ß-hemolytic streptococci (among others), acute bacterial endocarditis (ABE). Both result from a bacteremia. ABE develops on normal valves and causes fenestration (perforation) of valve cusps and septic embolism and infarction, because the causative organisms are highly virulent. Embolism and infarction in SBE are usually bland. Focal ("embolic") glomerulonephritis occurs in SBE, probably on an immunologic basis. The verrucae on heart valves in terminal illnesses are sterile. Valvular prostheses are more often the site of ABE than SBE.

Rheumatic fever (RF) is a recurring febrile illness, more frequent in children than in adults and having a tendency to involve the heart and joints. Group A ß-hemolytic streptococci are causally related. Patients with rheumatic fever show a high frequency of antistreptolysin O. There is a cross-reaction between streptococcal hyaluronate and glycoproteins of valvular tissue and of streptococcal M-protein with cardiac myocytes.

In most instances the clinical syndrome of acute rheumatic fever follows an infection due to streptococcus group A. Usually the streptococcal infection subsides, and about 2 to 4 weeks later there is recurrence of fever, often with migratory joint pain and swelling. Leukocytosis and an increased erythrocyte sedimentation rate are commonly noted. Involuntary muscle movements (chorea), subcutaneous nodules, and a skin rash (erythema marginatum) occur in some cases.

Of the pathologic changes in the heart in acute rheumatic fever, the earliest visible lesions are on the valves, particularly the mitral valve. Tiny warty deposits, composed of fibrin, platelets, a few red cells, and leukocytes, are laid down in a row corresponding to the line of closure of the valves. Following single attacks there may be complete healing of the verrucae, without deformity. In other cases these exudative lesions are invaded at their base by fibroblasts. There is agglutination of the valve cusps at their commissures, and thickening and rigidity of the leaflets. With recurrences there is renewed exudation, followed again by organization and further deformity. Residual damage after rheumatic fever is a result of this deformity. Thickening, fusion, and shortening of the chordae tendineae of the mitral valve lead to mitral insufficiency. Rigidity and fusion of the cusps lead to mitral stenosis.

During the active febrile phase of rheumatic fever, the myocardium is usually involved. Aschoff bodies occur along the course of small vessels and are most numerous in the myocardium of the left ventricle. The Aschoff body is a focal lesion consisting of fragments of muscle fibers and strands of collagen and fibrinoid material intermingled with large histiocytes having multiple nuclei each with a central chromatin mass, making the nucleus appear like an owl's eye (Aschoff cells). Anitschkow myocytes, which are spindle-shaped and have a longitudinal chromatin bar in the nucleus (caterpillar nucleus), are often numerous. Acute pericarditis occurs in acute rheumatic fever. There is a serofibrinous or fibrinous inflammation of the pericardium.

Joint lesions, commonly in the knees, are usually transient. During an acute attack the synovia is edematous and infiltrated with mononuclear cells and fibrinoid deposits. Subcutaneous nodules are often found along extensor tendons on extremities. They show a large central focus of fibrinoid necrosis. Erythema marginatum usually appears on the trunk as maculopapules. The centers tend to clear as the lesions enlarge.

Mitral stenosis is the classic residual valvular lesion after recurrent rheumatic fever. The stenosis is due to thickening and rigidity of the cusps, and agglutination of the cusps at the commissures. Mitral stenosis is more common in females than in males. Functionally there is interference with filling of the left ventricle, hence reduction of left ventricular output during systole. In addition, there are hypertrophy and dilatation of the left atrium, engorgement of the pulmonary circulation (pulmonary hypertension), and right ventricular hypertrophy. Thrombosis may occur in the left atrial appendix, especially when atrial fibrillation develops. This may result in embolism in the systemic circulation.

Mitral insufficiency is a very common clinical diagnosis but difficult to recognize at necropsy except in association with mitral stenosis. Shortening of the chordae tendineae or dilatation of the left ventricle may hold the mitral orifice open during ventricular systole. Insufficiency may also be caused by widening of the mitral annulus and papillary muscle dysfunction. The effect of mitral insufficiency is a leakage of blood from the left ventricle back into the left atrium during systole, thereby reducing the systolic output into the aorta. Hypertrophy and dilatation of both the left atrium and the left ventricle result.

Aortic stenosis is among the valvular heart diseases second in importance only to mitral stenosis. In some instances the cusps are thickened and agglutinated at their commissures, but are not nodular or distorted. More often the cusps show nodular calcified masses, distorting the commissures, narrowing the orifice and rendering the cusps more rigid. In calcific aortic valve disease the male to female ratio is about 4 to 1. Calcific aortic stenosis may be a result of rheumatic fever or a sequela of chronic bacterial endocarditis or a congenitally bicuspid aortic valve.

The effect of aortic stenosis is to interfere with the systolic ejection of blood from the left ventricle; marked hypertrophy of the left ventricle results. Sudden death without prior symptoms may be due to heart block (the conduction bundle may be compressed by the calcified masses at the base of the aortic valve) or to the sudden onset of coronary insufficiency when left ventricular failure begins. Conduction defects, including complete heart block, are commonly observed on the electrocardiogram.

Aortic insufficiency may be due to extension of an inflammatory reaction from the aorta, with shortening and rolling of the cusps and widening of the commissures, as in syphilis; to thickening and retraction of the cusps, as in rheumatic fever; to congenital or acquired dilatation of the aortic valve ring; or to nodular calcific lesions of the cusps, like those seen in calcific aortic stenosis except that the orifice is held rigidly open. The effect of aortic insufficiency is to add a great burden to the left ventricle, since it must force out a greater than normal quantity of blood with each systole in order to compensate for the valvular leakage. Marked hypertrophy of the left ventricle results.

Floppy valve syndrome (Barlow's syndrome) often occurs in women 20-40 years of age. There is a striking familial incidence. The cause is unknown, but it may represent a localized form of Marfan's syndrome. Myxomatous degeneration of valve leaflets also occurs in elderly persons, especially men, probably due to a degenerative aging process.

Grossly in the floppy valve syndrome, there may be slight left ventricular hypertrophy. The mitral valve circumference is increased, and its leaflets are thickened and redundant. The posterior leaflet is usually more severely involved and balloons into the left atrial chamber. The leaflets are pearly gray and glistening. The chordae tendineae are long and thin and occasionally rupture. Microscopically, focal myxomatous degeneration is found in the thickened valve leaflets.

Acute endocarditis usually occurs as a complication of a bacterial or mycotic infection in some other part of the body, and the causative agent is usually Staphylococcus aureus, ß-hemolytic streptococci, Escherichia coli, Pseudomonas aeruginosa, and other gram-negative organisms, and fungi such as Candida. Endocarditis is common among drug addicts and diabetics. Fungal and bacterial infections occasionally occur on valve prostheses.

The aortic and mitral valves are most commonly affected, especially if these valves are already abnormal, as from rheumatic fever or a congenital defect, Normal valves may also be involved. The affected valve usually shows evidence of extensive destruction, often with perforation. Vegetations are usually massive and friable. The lytic action of the bacterial and leukocytic enzymes results in frequent, often massive, septic emboli.

Subacute bacterial endocarditis (SBE) is usually a slowly developing febrile illness. In most instances the avenue of entry of the infecting organism is not evident. Occasionally onset is preceded by dental extraction, cystoscopy, or some other type of manipulation. The causative agent is usually the α-hemolytic group of streptococci (S. viridans).

The disease occurs as a late complication of valvular heart disease, usually rheumatic or congenital. The frequency of involvement of valves is mitral, aortic, and tricuspid. The affected valve may show evidence of previous rheumatic disease: fibrosis, thickening, and agglutination of the cusps. In addition, small, firm, vegetations composed of fibrin, a few leukocytes, and bacteria are attached to the surface of the valves. The organisms tend to cause a slow dissolution of the vegetations, small bits breaking off at a time. The myocardium often shows minute abscesses (Bracht-Wächter lesions). Infarcts are found in various organs. Although the emboli may contain bacteria, the resulting infarcts do not suppurate. In the kidneys, a focal ("embolic") glomerulonephritis with foci of fibrinoid necrosis in glomerular tufts may occur. It is probably due to immune complex deposition.

159. The causes of myocarditis include all of the following **EXCEPT**:

    (A) Coxsackie virus group B infection
    (B) diphtheria exotoxin
    (C) Chagas' disease
    (D) syphilis
    (E) toxoplasmosis

160. Drugs which cause hypersensitivity myocarditis include all of the following **EXCEPT**:

    (A) ampicillin
    (B) furosemide
    (C) lovastatin
    (D) methyldopa
    (E) sulfonamides

161. An 18 year-old boy developed dull chest pain, dyspnea, and a pericardial friction rub. The causes of fibrinous pericarditis include all of the following **EXCEPT**:

    (A) Coxsackie virus group B infection
    (B) diphtheria exotoxin
    (C) myocardial infarction
    (D) rheumatic heart disease
    (E) uremia

162. Of the following constrictive pericarditis is most likely to be due to

    (A) Coxsackie virus group B infection
    (B) metastatic carcinoma
    (C) rheumatic heart disease
    (D) tuberculosis
    (E) uremia

163. An 18 year-old basketball player collapsed on the court and died. Of the following the likeliest cause is

    (A) acute myocardial infarction
    (B) dilated (congestive) cardiomyopathy
    (C) floppy valve syndrome with rupture of chordae tendineae
    (D) hypertrophic cardiomyopathy
    (E) rheumatic myocarditis

164. Causative factors which have been used to explain the development of dilated (congestive) cardiomyopathy include all of the following **EXCEPT**:

    (A) chronic alcoholism
    (B) cobalt formerly used in beer
    (C) inheritance as an autosomal dominant
    (D) nutritional deficiency in pregnancy
    (E) viral myocarditis

165. Pathologic findings in idiopathic hypertrophic subaortic stenosis include all of the following **EXCEPT**:

    (A) infiltration of eosinophils in myocardium
    (B) myocardial fiber disorientation in interventricular septum
    (C) thickening of anterior leaflet of mitral valve
    (D) thickening of septum greater than of free wall of left ventricle
    (E) small ventricular cavities

166. Infiltrative (restrictive) cardiomyopathy occurs in all of the following **EXCEPT**:

    (A) amyloidosis
    (B) Gaucher's disease
    (C) glycogen storage disease
    (D) hemochromatosis
    (E) sarcoidosis

ANSWERS AND TUTORIAL ON ITEMS 159-166

The answers are: **159-D; 160-C; 161-B; 162-D; 163-D; 164-C; 165-A; 166-B**. Myocarditis signifies inflammation of the myocardium. Rheumatic myocarditis is the most common type and occurs during the course of acute rheumatic fever. Interstitial myocarditis, characterized by focal collections of lymphocytes and macrophages about small vessels, may be seen in fatal cases of many infectious diseases, including varicella, diphtheria, scarlet fever, typhoid fever, and group B Coxsackie viral infections. Myocarditis also occurs in toxoplasmosis and Chagas' disease (due to Trypanosoma cruzi). Hypersensitivity myocarditis due to drugs such as methyldopa, sulfonamides, ampicillin, and furosemide, is characterized by an infiltration of eosinophils, macrophages, and predominantly T-lymphocytes.

Acute pericarditis usually follows infection of some other organ. Suppurative pericarditis is usually a complication of bacteremia or spread from an adjacent pleuritis. Tuberculous pericarditis is usually due to spread to the pericardial sac from adjacent tuberculous lymph nodes. Rheumatic pericarditis may occur along with rheumatic endocarditis and myocarditis.

Pericarditis occurs in uremia, myocardial infarction, and viral infections, especially Coxsackie B.

In acute pericarditis due to pyogenic bacteria, the fluid is frankly purulent. In nonspecific pericarditis and in pericarditis due to rheumatic fever, the fluid is sterile, usually slightly cloudy, and contains fibrin. In tuberculous pericarditis, there may be frank caseation necrosis of the involved tissues and a thick layer of fibrin may collect, or there may be a blood-tinged effusion. In pericarditis due to myocardial infarction, fibrin is commonly deposited over the necrotic area of the myocardium. In uremic pericarditis, a dry fibrinous exudate is usual.

Adhesions of minor degree are often encountered between the two layers of the pericardium. When pericardial adhesions are thick, and particularly when they are associated with mediastinal, pleural, and chest wall adhesions, they may produce heart failure. Constrictive pericarditis (Pick's disease) is a sequel of mediastinal tuberculosis. Dense scar tissue, often with a heavy layer of calcium frosting, may surround the ventricles, atria, or great vessels as an unyielding band. As a result the heart chambers may be unable to dilate to receive blood during diastole.

A cardiomyopathy is a non-inflammatory disorder in which the involvement is primarily in the myocardium. It may be classified as idiopathic, infiltrative, or endomyocardial in type. The idiopathic form is divided into dilated and nondilated (hypertrophic) types. In the latter, the hypertrophy may be symmetric or asymmetric.

Dilated (congestive) cardiomyopathy occurs in men more often than in women and is frequently associated with chronic alcoholism (possibly due to an associated thiamine deficiency). Cobalt formerly added to beer was a causative factor. It may also be related to nutritional deficiency in pregnancy and the post partum period. Doxorubicin therapy and viral myocarditis have also been implicated. The average heart weight is 600 gms. The left ventricular wall is usually less than 1.5 cm. thick. The myocardium is flabby. All four cardiac chambers are dilated. Recent and old thrombi are often present in the ventricles and atrial appendages, and embolism is common. Death is usually due to congestive heart failure.

In symmetric hypertrophic cardiomyopathy the heart is enlarged, averaging over 600 gms., and the left ventricular myocardium is more than 1.5 cm. thick. The interventricular septum is similar in thickness to the ventricular free wall, and ventricular outflow obstruction does not occur. Asymmetric hypertrophic cardiomyopathy is more common than the symmetric type and is usually associated with ventricular outlet obstruction (idiopathic hypertrophic subaortic stenosis, IHSS). It is transmitted as an autosomal dominant. In IHSS, the septal myocardium is thicker than the free wall. The ventricular cavities are small (muscle bound heart), and the atria are dilated. There is thickening of the mitral valve, and a plaque forms on the septal endocardium where it is slapped by the anterior leaflet of the mitral valve. Microscopically, the myocardial fibers of the septum are disoriented, running in all directions rather than parallel to each other. Hypertrophic cardiomyopathy often occurs in young adults and may lead to sudden death during athletic activity or strenuous exercise.

Infiltrative (restrictive) cardiomyopathy may occur in amyloidosis, sarcoidosis, hemochromatosis (iron deposition), glycogen storage disease types II, III and IV, and Fabry's disease (glycolipid deposition).

Items 167-179

In Items 167-174, match the pathologic changes with the stage or stages of atherosclerosis in which each occurs typically.

        (A)   fibrous plaque
        (B)   complicated plaque
        (C)   both
        (D)   neither

167. atheroma formation

168. calcium deposits in intima

169. calcium deposits in media

170. cholesterol deposits

171. fatty streak

172. increase in myointimal cells

173. thrombosis on surface

174. ulceration of surface

175. Complications of atherosclerosis of the aorta include all of the following **EXCEPT**:

        (A)   aneurysm formation
        (B)   atheroembolism
        (C)   bacterial endaortitis
        (D)   leiomyoma (smooth muscle tumor) formation
        (E)   thromboembolism

176. A 50 year-old man had angina on slight exertion. An angiogram revealed partial obstruction of all 3 main coronary arteries. All of the following are major risk factors for the development of coronary artery disease **EXCEPT**:

        (A)   cigarette smoking
        (B)   diabetes mellitus
        (C)   hypercholesterolemia
        (D)   hypertension
        (E)   obesity

177. A 60 year-old man who had been diagnosed 3 days before as having had an acute myocardial infarct suddenly developed mitral insufficiency. This was most likely due to

   (A)   coincidental rheumatic mitral stenosis
   (B)   extension of the infarct to a mitral valve leaflet
   (C)   rupture of an infarcted interventricular septum
   (D)   rupture of an infarcted papillary muscle
   (E)   subacute bacterial endocarditis on the mitral valve

A 65 year-old man died of what was diagnosed clinically as an acute myocardial infarct. It was confirmed at autopsy grossly. A photograph and photomicrograph of the lesion are shown in Figure 2.1.

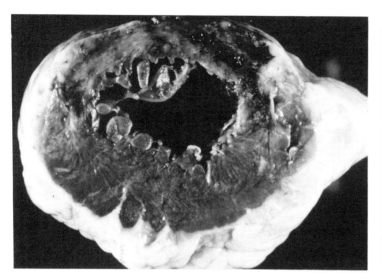 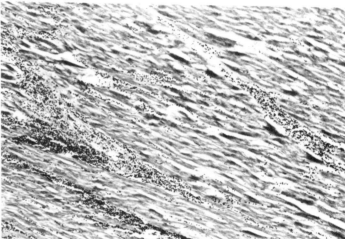

Figure 2.1

178.   The approximate age of this myocardial infarct from the time of onset of chest pain is

(A)   12 hours
(B)   24 hours
(C)   3 days
(D)   7 days
(E)   10 days

179.   The most frequent cause of acute myocardial infarction is occlusion of a major coronary artery by

(A)   atherosclerosis
(B)   embolism
(C)   spasm
(D)   subintimal hemorrhage
(E)   thrombosis

ANSWERS AND TUTORIAL ON ITEMS 167-179

The answers are: **167-C; 168-B; 169-D; 170-C; 171-D; 172-A; 173-B; 174-B; 175-D; 176-E; 177-D; 178-C; 179-E.**

> Atheroma is the generic name for both types of plaque. The fatty streak occurs in children and disappears later in life. The fibrous plaque is formed by accumulation of cholesterol and other lipids and collagen laid down by myointimal cells which have entered the intima from the media. Calcium deposits in the intima, cholesterol, ulceration of the endothelial surface, and thrombosis all occur in a complicated plaque. Calcification of the media occurs in Mönckeberg's sclerosis and is not related to atherosclerosis. As to complications of atherosclerosis, although myointimal cells participate in formation of plaque, they do not produce smooth muscle tumors.
>
> Of the risk factors for coronary (and other) atherosclerosis, obesity alone is probably not a primary cause. However, it is frequently associated with other risk factors. Rupture of an infarcted papillary muscle allows a mitral cusp to fly free and produce mitral insufficiency. The infarct in the photomicrograph shows the degree of coagulation necrosis and leukocyte infiltration found in one about 3 days old. No or little change is apparent in the first day, and by a week granulation tissue would be present. In about two thirds of cases of acute MI, a thrombus is found in the atherosclerotic artery supplying the infarcted zone.

The weight of evidence seems to favor the view that a site of atherosclerosis develops as a reaction to endothelial injury. Increased permeability allows plasma proteins, including lipoproteins, to enter the intima. Adherent platelets, macrophages, and endothelial cells elaborate growth factors which stimulate proliferation of medial smooth muscle cells. These then migrate into the intima and synthesize collagen. Lipids accumulate within these myointimal cells and macrophages (foam cells) and extracellularly.

Minimal lesions of atherosclerosis (fibrous plaques) are evident grossly as raised yellowish plaques. Microscopically, there is an increase in the collagen and other ground substance of the intima (fibrous cap). Smooth muscle (myointimal) cells are increased in number. Fine droplets of lipid in the intimal tissues, sometimes in foam cells (lipophages), may be noted. In larger lesions lipid masses coalesce, intervening tissues disintegrate and even liquefy, and cholesterol crystals appear. At this stage the lesion is soft, and elevated above the surrounding intima (an atheroma).

Larger complicated plaques tend to attract calcium into their substance by the process of dystrophic calcification. When calcium is added in sufficient amount, the plaque becomes hard and inelastic. Atheromatous ulcers and surface thrombi are common. Depending upon the size of the vessel affected and the direction of the forces involved, a thrombus may form, closing the vessel, or the elevated plaque may itself close a small artery (such as a coronary) effectively.

In large arteries, such as the aorta, atheromatous lesions cause no significant narrowing of the lumen. In the cerebral or coronary arteries or the arteries of the lower extremities, there is narrowing of the lumen by the atheromatous plaques. Ischemia of the affected part often follows. In arteries of any size the vessel may be weakened at the site of an atheroma, resulting in thinning of the wall and predisposing to aneurysm formation, rupture, and hemorrhage. The roughened intima predisposes to thrombus formation.

The clinical manifestations in atherosclerosis are dependent upon the effects of the atheromatous plaque itself (i.e., narrowing of the arterial lumen and ischemia of the affected part) and upon the local developments in or on atheromatous lesions (hemorrhage or thrombosis). Ischemia is usually manifested by a gradual impairment of function, while hemorrhage or thrombosis is usually revealed by sudden catastrophic symptoms related to the affected part. Atheromatous embolism results from the spontaneous breaking off of portions of an atheromatous plaque, usually from the aorta. The emboli may lodge in small arteries of the brain, spleen, kidneys, or other organs and cause infarction. The presence of cholesterol clefts and other components of atheromata identify the emboli. Rarely during a bacteremia organisms may localize on a plaque, causing an endaortitis. An aneurysm may occur with severe atherosclerosis, especially in the abdominal aorta. Rupture of an atherosclerotic aneurysm may cause an exsanguinating hemorrhage.

Coronary artery disease (ischemic heart disease) (IHD), like atherosclerosis in general, is intimately related to cholesterol metabolism, blood coagulation, and fibrinolysis. The major coronary risk factors are hypercholesterolemia, cigarette smoking, and hypertension. Diabetes mellitus and being male are also important risk factors.

Occlusion of a coronary artery results from thrombosis in about two-thirds of the cases, but it may follow a tear in the coronary intima adjacent to a plaque, permitting blood to dissect the plaque upward by subintimal hemorrhage. Occasionally a coronary artery is occluded as a result of embolism, as in bacterial endocarditis. When coronary occlusion is due to thrombosis, it usually occurs at a point of narrowing of the artery by atherosclerosis. Ulceration of a plaque leads to surface breaks on which platelets are deposited. Fibrin then forms on the platelet coagulum, and cellular elements of blood are enmeshed to form the thrombus. In some cases coronary occlusion causing myocardial ischemia and even infarction has been attributed to coronary arterial spasm.

The anterior descending branch of the left coronary artery is the vessel which usually shows the greatest evidence of atherosclerosis and has the highest frequency of thrombotic occlusion. Corresponding infarcts occur at the apex and anterior wall of the left ventricle, and especially in the apical portion of the interventricular septum. Occlusion of the right coronary artery or the circumflex branch of the left coronary artery usually causes infarction of the posterior or lateral wall of the left ventricle. Infarction of the right ventricle or of either atrium is rare.

In the area of myocardial ischemia, certain chemical changes precede the development of visible lesions: a decrease in muscle glycogen and a disappearance of the cardiac muscle enzymes, creatine phosphokinase (CPK), aspartate aminotransferase (AST), and lactic dehydrogenase (LDH). As these enzymes disappear from the infarcted muscle, values for them rise markedly in the serum. Morphologic changes follow these chemical changes. An hour or two after experimental occlusion, the regular myofibrillar pattern is disrupted by a foamy cytoplasmic change, contraction bands are prominent, fibers become separated by edema fluid. Beginning about the fourth hour after onset, the cell cytoplasm undergoes striking changes leading to protein coagulation, followed by nuclear changes of necrosis. After about 24 hours, leukocytes begin to invade the infarct from the periphery. After 2 days the infarct appears grossly as a yellowish area with hemorrhagic borders. If the infarct extends to the endocardial or epicardial surface, fibrin will form on the surface. A mural thrombus may form over the area of infarction. Fibrin on the surface of the epicardium may lead to the development of a pericardial friction rub. As a result of lytic action of the leukocytic enzymes, dead muscle fibers are broken up, beginning about 5 days after thrombosis. Fibroblasts proliferate, collagen is laid down, and a scar is formed. Stretching of the scar is common, due to inelasticity, and an old infarct is usually marked by a thin, white area of outpouching of the ventricular wall. If this is extreme, the lesion is an aneurysm of the heart.

If the patient survives the hypotensive phase of the first few days, a second critical period is sometimes noted 5 to 12 days after the onset. At this time, corresponding to the phase of softening and lysis of the infarct, rupture of the ventricle may occur, with the tear extending through the wall, resulting in hemopericardium and cardiac tamponade. More rarely the tear may be through the interventricular septum, producing an intracardiac shunt, or through a papillary muscle, leading to mitral insufficiency.

Items 180-188

180. The manifestations of syphilitic cardiovascular disease include all of the following **EXCEPT**:

    (A)   aneurysm of the ascending aorta
    (B)   aortitis
    (C)   aortic valvular insufficiency
    (D)   cystic medial necrosis of aorta
    (E)   narrowing of coronary ostia

181. A 75 year-old man went into shock and collapsed suddenly. He died shortly after reaching the hospital. A ruptured abdominal aortic aneurysm was found. The most common cause of such an aneurysm is

    (A)   atherosclerosis
    (B)   bacterial infection
    (C)   developmental defect
    (D)   tertiary syphilis
    (E)   trauma

182. Complications of aortic aneurysms include all of the following **EXCEPT**:

    (A)   erosion of bones
    (B)   pulmonary embolism
    (C)   rupture with cardiac tamponade
    (D)   rupture with exsanguination
    (E)   thrombosis in sac

183. Dissecting aneurysm of the aorta is associated with all of the following **EXCEPT**:

   (A) cystic medial necrosis
   (B) hypertension
   (C) rupture with cardiac tamponade
   (D) Marfan's syndrome
   (E) syphilis

184. The causes of cor pulmonale include all of the following **EXCEPT**:

   (A) emphysema of the lungs
   (B) interventricular septal defect (late)
   (C) kyphoscoliosis
   (D) lung abscess
   (E) recurrent pulmonary embolism

185. The commonest primary neoplasm of the heart is the

   (A) lipoma
   (B) myxoma
   (C) papillary fibroelastoma
   (D) rhabdomyoma
   (E) rhabdomyosarcoma

186. The commonest site of metastatic neoplasm in the heart is the

   (A) endocardium
   (B) myocardium
   (C) pericardium
   (D) right atrium
   (E) valve cusps

187. The malignant neoplasms which most commonly give rise to cardiac metastases include all of the following **EXCEPT**:

   (A) bronchogenic carcinoma
   (B) carcinoma of the breast
   (C) carcinoma of the thyroid gland
   (D) lymphomas
   (E) malignant melanoma

72

188. Conditions associated with intracardiac thrombosis and arterial embolism include all of the following **EXCEPT**:

   (A)   dilated (congestive) cardiomyopathy
   (B)   mitral stenosis
   (C)   myocardial infarction
   (D)   subacute bacterial endocarditis
   (E)   viral myocarditis

ANSWERS AND TUTORIAL ON ITEMS 180-188

The answers are: **180-D; 181-A; 182-B; 183-E; 184-D; 185-B; 186-C; 187-C; 188-E**. Many forms of syphilis of the cardiovascular system have their beginnings in syphilitic aortitis. The interval between the appearance of the chancre and clinical evidence of syphilitic aortitis is usually 5 to 15 years. The spirochete has an affinity for the ascending and transverse limbs of the aortic arch. Grossly, the affected portion of the aorta is somewhat dilated. Syphilitic fibrosis of the media, with destruction of muscularis and elastica, results in puckered stellate depressions of the intima, separated by wrinkled areas. The aorta is greatly weakened. Microscopically, the media shows scattered foci of necrosis and fibrous scarring. The adventitia and outer portion of media show perivascular infiltration by plasma cells and lymphocytes. The vasa vasorum show luminal narrowing due to endarteritis obliterans.

Insufficiency of the aortic valve results when the syphilitic fibrosis of the aortic media spreads to the commissures of the aortic valve, separating one cusp from another, and causing thickening, shortening, and rolling of the cusp edges. Left ventricular dilatation and hypertrophy develop and often become extreme. Coronary insufficiency is an important although uncommon complication of syphilitic aortitis. When the inflammatory fibrosis of the aortic wall happens to surround one or both coronary ostia, the scarring may narrow the lumen sufficiently to cause symptoms. Sudden death is common in such cases.

Any localized dilatation of the lumen of a blood vessel is a true aneurysm. A false aneurysm is a localized external widening of a vessel without dilatation of the lumen, often due to a hematoma between its layers.

Most aneurysms occur in the aorta or its major branches, often at a localized area of weakening in the vessel wall. Atherosclerosis and medial dissection are the major causes. All aneurysms are more common in males. When rupture occurs, it may cause exsanguinating hemorrhage, or the accumulation of blood may so compress vital structures such as the heart due to intrapericardial hemorrhage (cardiac tamponade) as to cause death. When an aneurysm of an intracranial artery ruptures, it usually causes death by increased intracranial pressure due to subarachnoid hemorrhage.

Atherosclerosis is the most frequent cause of aortic aneurysm. In most instances, the affected patients are males in the seventh or eighth decade. The abdominal aorta, generally below the renal arteries, is the most common site. The iliac arteries are the next most frequent sites of atherosclerotic aneurysm development.

Atheromatous lesions weaken the affected vessels and, when combined with loss of elastica in the media, result in dilatation. An unruptured arteriosclerotic aneurysm of the abdominal aorta often causes no symptoms. When rupture occurs, it is usually into the retroperitoneal tissues, where a mass appears and enlarges over a period of a few hours. Exsanguination is the usual end result, but many patients are saved by surgical excision of the aneurysm and replacement with a graft or prosthesis.

A dissecting aneurysm (dissecting hematoma) is a form of false aneurysm in which there is a splitting of the media of the aorta, usually at the juncture of the inner two thirds and outer third. Blood enters the split and extends it, resulting in an elongated hematoma in the wall. Most patients with dissecting aneurysm have a long history of severe hypertension. Some patients with dissecting aneurysm show evidence of Marfan's syndrome. Zones of medial necrosis, sometimes associated with small, slitlike cysts (medial cystic necrosis of Erdheim), are often found in aortas showing dissecting aneurysm.

"Congenital" (berry) aneurysm occurs on or near the circle of Willis, especially the anterior communicating artery, the middle or anterior cerebral arteries, or the basilar artery, usually at or near a point of bifurcation, where the media is thin normally. About 30 percent develop on the anterior, middle and posterior cerebral arteries respectively and 10 percent on the basilar and vertebral arteries. "Congenital" aneurysms are saccular in form and vary from 0.1 to 3 cm. in diameter. The wall of the aneurysm is composed of a greatly thickened intima, with complete absence of the media and internal elastic lamina. With rupture or leakage of the aneurysm, subarachnoid hemorrhage develops. Bright red blood floods the subarachnoid space.

Cor pulmonale signifies right ventricular strain. As the term is generally used it implies a chronic disorder, associated with right ventricular hypertrophy. Acute cor pulmonale is the term for the sudden right ventricular strain that is a sequel to massive pulmonary embolism.

Primary obstruction to pulmonary blood flow may be due to stenosis of the pulmonic valve; conditions which block blood flow in major pulmonary arteries (recurring pulmonary embolism), or in pulmonary arterioles (idiopathic pulmonary hypertension; left-to-right shunts due to septal defects or persistent ductus arteriosus); or stenosis of the mitral valve orifice.

Primary difficulty in ventilation may result from emphysema (about 80 percent of cases), pulmonary fibrosis, or diseases restricting thoracic mobility (kyphoscoliosis, extreme obesity). Patients with these conditions show cyanosis and dyspnea, and examination reveals thoracic deformity and expiratory wheezes. Cor pulmonale results from pulmonary vasoconstriction due to hypoxia and respiratory acidosis and from the development of bronchopulmonary vascular shunts.

Primary neoplasms of the heart are rare and are usually benign. Myxoma is the most common primary neoplasm. It is a soft mass, consisting of edematous connective tissue irregularly covered by thrombus, commonly attached to the endocardium by a pedicle, and hanging free into a cavity, usually the left atrium. It may block the mitral orifice, producing a murmur like that of mitral stenosis. Embolism from the surface of the neoplasm or an overlying thrombus is common. The papillary fibroelastoma is very rare and occurs on heart valves. Rhabdomyoma (which is associated with tuberous sclerosis) and rhabdomyosarcoma are extremely rare neoplasms arising in cardiac muscles cells in children. Metastatic neoplasms of the heart, especially in the pericardium, are fairly common. The neoplasms commonly giving rise to cardiac metastases are those primary to the breasts and lungs, as well as lymphomas and melanomas.

CHAPTER III

HEMATOLOGICAL AND LYMPHATIC PATHOLOGY
IMMUNOPATHOLOGY

Items 189-203

In Items 189-196, match each clinical summary with the type of anemia with which it is most closely related.

     (A) α-thalassemia
     (B)   anemia due to glucose-6-phosphate dehydrogenase deficiency
     (C)   aplastic anemia
     (D)   autoimmune hemolytic anemia
     (E)   ß-thalassemia
     (F)   hereditary spherocytic anemia
     (G)   iron deficiency anemia
     (H)   myelophthisic anemia
     (I)   pernicious anemia
     (J)   sickle cell anemia
     (K)   sideroblastic anemia

189.   A 10 year-old boy was found to have mild jaundice, with an elevation mainly of unconjugated bilirubin, and splenomegaly. His erythrocyte count was 4 million/mm^3 and the red cells showed increased fragility in hypotonic saline.

190.   A 4 year-old African-American child developed pneumonia. While being treated he began to have episodes of bone pain. His erythrocyte count was 3 million/mm^3, and the corrected reticulocyte count was 3%. The serum iron was 120 μg/dL.

191.   An Italian-American child was noted to be listless, easily fatigued, and pale. His erythrocyte count was 2 million/mm^3, corrected reticulocyte count 5%, and serum iron 100 μg/dL. Numerous target cells were seen on the peripheral blood smear. HbF and HbA$_2$ were present in significant amounts.

192.   A 25 year-old woman had menometrorrhagia for several months. She complained of being weak and chronically tired. Her erythrocyte count was 3.5 million/mm^3, corrected reticulocyte count 1%, and serum iron 50 μg/dL with a high total iron binding capacity.

193. A 60 year-old man gave a 6 month history of gradually worsening fatigue and dyspnea on exertion. He had tingling in his feet. His erythrocyte count was 2 million/mm^3. Gastric analysis revealed achlorhydria.

194. A 65 year-old woman with a history of a mastectomy for breast cancer 2 years before suffered collapse of several vertebrae. She was found to have extensive bony metastases. Her erythrocyte count was 3 million/mm^3 and corrected reticulocyte count 1%.

195. A 40 year-old woman developed weakness, pallor, skin hemorrhages, and fever. Her erythrocyte count was 1.5 million/mm^3, leukocyte count 1500/mm^3, and platelet count 40,000/mm^3.

196. A 40 year-old African-American Viet Nam veteran developed episodes of hemolysis on using certain drugs. Numerous Heinz bodies were found in his erythrocytes during these periods.

197. Pathologic changes in patients with sickle cell anemia may include all of the following **EXCEPT**:

    (A)   bilirubin gallstones
    (B)   fat and bone marrow embolism
    (C)   infarcts in bones and spleen
    (D)   priapism
    (E)   tendency to develop acute leukemia

198. The presence of HbF in the blood of children and adults is characteristic of

    (A)   α-thalassemia
    (B)   ß-thalassemia
    (C)   megaloblastic anemia
    (D)   sickle cell anemia
    (E)   spherocytic anemia

199. Autoimmune hemolytic anemia occurs in all of the following **EXCEPT**:

    (A)   chronic lymphocytic leukemia
    (B)   patients on methyldopa therapy
    (C)   patients on penicillin therapy
    (D)   polyarteritis nodosa
    (E)   systemic lupus erythematosus

200. The commonest cause of iron deficiency anemia in adults in the United States is

(A) chronic blood loss
(B) chronic renal failure
(C) inadequate iron intake in diet
(D) iron loss due to hemolysis
(E) mucosal block to iron absorption in duodenum

201. Pathologic changes in pernicious anemia include all of the following **EXCEPT**:

(A) atrophic gastritis
(B) degeneration of posterior columns and pyramidal tracts in spinal cord
(C) esophageal web
(D) leukopenia with multisegmented neutrophils
(E) macrocytes in peripheral blood

202. Myelophthisic anemia due to bone marrow replacement occurs in all of the following **EXCEPT**:

(A) leukemia
(B) lipid storage diseases
(C) multiple myeloma
(D) myelofibrosis
(E) Waldenström's macroglobulinemia

203. The causes of aplastic anemia include all of the following **EXCEPT**:

(A) benzene
(B) chloramphenicol
(C) cancer chemotherapeutic agents
(D) penicillin
(E) phenylbutazone

ANSWERS AND TUTORIAL ON ITEMS 189-203

The answers are: **189-F; 190-J; 191-E; 192-G; 193-I; 194-H; 195-C; 196-B; 197-E; 198-B; 199-D; 200-A; 201-C; 202-E; 203-D**.

In Item 189, hemolysis, splenomegaly, and increased osmotic fragility of erythrocytes point to congenital spherocytic anemia.

In Item 190, the triggering of a crisis by pneumonia and the bone pain in an African American child are indicative of sickle cell anemia.

In Item 191, severe anemia with target cells and HbF and HbA$_2$ in this child is indicative of ß-thalassemia.

In Item 192, chronic blood loss has led to iron depletion and anemia, which is corroborated by the low serum iron and high iron binding capacity.

In Item 193, the tingling of the feet, achlorhydria, and severe anemia are characteristic of pernicious anemia.

In Item 194, extensive bony metastases lead to a diagnosis of myelophthic anemia.

In Item 195, the presence of anemia, leukopenia, and thrombocytopenia are indicative of aplastic anemia.

In Item 196, hemolysis on use of an antimalarial drug and Heinz bodies occur with G-6-PD deficiency in erythrocytes.

Anemia is an abnormally low value for circulating RBCs and hemoglobin per unit volume of blood with impairment of oxygen delivery to body cells.

Hereditary spherocytosis is transmitted as an autosomal dominant. There is hemolysis with jaundice, splenic enlargement, spherocytosis, and increased RBC fragility in hypotonic saline solution. The spherocytes are destroyed excessively in the spleen. The basic cause appears to be a defect in spectrin, a filamentous protein important in maintaining RBC membrane stability.

Congenital non-spherocytic hemolytic anemias are due to a hereditary deficiency of an erythrocyte enzyme. The most important is glucose-6-phosphate dehydrogenase (G-6-PD) deficiency in erythrocytes, which is transmitted as a sex-linked characteristic. A few men with the trait have a chronic hemolytic anemia without challenge. Most develop hemolysis only after ingestion of fava beans or a drug such as primaquine. Numerous Heinz bodies, consisting of denatured hemoglobin, appear in erythrocytes in G-6-PD deficiency.

Sickle cell anemia is transmitted homozygously as recessive trait and is characterized by sickling of red cells under reduced oxygen tension. It is a hemoglobinopathy. Hemoglobin S (HbS) differs from normal HbA by the substitution of valine for glutamic acid in its ß chains. Heterozygotes carry 35 to 45% HbS in their red cells. Homozygotes have 80 to 100%.

Pathologic changes in sickle cell anemia are largely caused by capillary stasis due to sickling. This may result in infarction in bones, small intestine, spleen, gray cortex, and retina, as well as priapism. Venous thrombosis and pulmonary embolism may occur, as well as fat and bone marrow embolism. Except in aplastic crisis the bone marrow shows erythroid hyperplasia. As a result of the repeated hemolytic episodes, hemosiderin deposits develop in the liver, spleen, bone marrow, and lymph nodes. Bilirubin gallstones are commonly found in the gallbladder.

Thalassemia (Mediterranean or Cooley's anemia) is a hemoglobinopathic anemia in children of Italian and Greek heritage due to partial or complete failure of formation of a globin chain in their erythrocytes. In α-thalassemia there is a gene deletion on chromosome 16, and in ß-thalassemia there is a defect on chromosome 11. Children in whom the trait is homozygous develop a severe anemia (thalassemia major). Those who are heterozygous have a mild anemia (thalassemia minor). In ß-thalassemia, beta chain formation is defective. HbA production is decreased, and there is increased formation of HbF (fetal hemoglobin) and HbA$_2$, which do not contain ß chains. The hemoglobin in erythrocytes contains an excess of α chains, which may be responsible for the hemolysis in ß-thalassemia.

Acquired hemolytic anemias are caused by chemical or bacterial agents, malarial parasites, heat (burns or heat stroke), or circulating autohemolysins. Autoimmune hemolytic anemia is due to the development of an immune reaction against erythrocytes. It usually occurs in cases of leukemia, lymphoma, or collagen vascular disease. Specific or nonspecific antigen-antibody complexes may bind to the erythrocyte plasma membrane in the presence of activated complement, producing hemolysis. Drug related immunohemolytic anemias may be of the haptene type (penicillin), immune complex type (quinidine), or true autoimmune type (methyldopa).

Iron deficiency anemia results from a chronic blood loss, an inadequate iron intake, or to interference with iron absorption in the intestine. The anemia is hypochromic and microcytic. In the bone marrow there is no stainable iron. Plummer-Vinson syndrome is iron deficiency anemia in middle-aged women together with atrophic glossitis, difficulty in swallowing due to an esophageal web, and spoon-shaped nails.

Megaloblastic anemia results from deficient absorption of vitamin B_{12} (cyanocobalamin) because of a deficiency of intrinsic factor in the gastric juice (pernicious anemia, PA) or some intestinal cause of malabsorption. Intrinsic factor is essential for B_{12} absorption. Diphyllobothrium latum (fish tapeworm) infestation and the blind loop syndrome in the small intestine may lead to a vitamin B_{12} deficiency. Megaloblastic anemia is also produced by a folic (pteryl-glutamic) acid deficiency. Folic acid absorption may be inhibited by diphenylhydantoin, methotrexate, 6-mercaptopurine, and 5-fluorouracil.

The deficiency of intrinsic factor is due to a congenital inability to form the factor in the childhood form of pernicious anemia. In 90 percent of adults with PA, there are serum antibodies against the cytoplasm of gastric parietal cells, which secrete intrinsic factor. There are also blocking and precipitating antibodies against intrinsic factor in almost all patients with pernicious anemia. During a relapse there is severe anemia with numerous macrocytes in the peripheral blood. There is also a leukopenia with a shift to the right (the presence of many multisegmented neutrophils). The deficiency of B_{12} or folic acid impairs DNA synthesis and cell division. Because of this the cells of the bone marrow and gastric and intestinal mucosa become abnormally large.

In a relapse in megaloblastic anemia the bone marrow contains many megaloblasts and normoblasts. The gastric fundus is thin, and the mucosa is atrophic (atrophic gastritis) in pernicious anemia. In the spinal cord, the posterior columns and pyramidal tracts show degeneration.

Myelophthisic anemia results from extensive marrow replacement in multiple myeloma, leukemia, metastatic carcinoma, lipid storage disease, or myelofibrosis (fibrous replacement).

Aplastic anemia is characterized by a severe decrease in or lack of erythropoietic, granulopoietic, and megakaryocytic bone marrow activity due to toxic inhibition. Causes include benzene, chloramphenicol, phenylbutazone, cancer chemotherapeutic agents, and ionizing radiation. In the peripheral blood, there is marked reduction in red and white cells and platelets. The bone marrow varies from moderate hematopoiesis to replacement by fat, fibrous tissue, or gelatinous material.

Items 204-212

204. A 40 year-old man who had been in good health developed headache and nuchal rigidity. A spinal tap confirmed the diagnosis of bacterial meningitis. He was also found to have anemia and thrombocytopenia. His white blood cell count was 30,000/mm$_3$. The blood smear showed very immature myeloid cells. The most likely diagnosis is

   (A)   acute myeloblastic leukemia
   (B)   acute promyelocytic leukemia
   (C)   aplastic anemia
   (D)   hairy cell leukemia
   (E)   leukemoid reaction

205. The most distinctive feature of acute myeloblastic leukemia is the presence of

   (A)   Auer bodies (eosinophilic rods) in myeloblasts
   (B)   blast crises
   (C)   chloromas
   (D)   Philadelphia chromosomes in neutrophils
   (E)   virus particles in myeloblasts

206. A 30 year-old woman presented with large hemorrhages in her skin, nosebleeds, and menometrorrhagia. Her white blood cell count was 35,000/mm^3 with numerous early myeloid cells on peripheral smear. The likeliest diagnosis is

   (A)   acute myeloblastic leukemia
   (B)   acute promyelocytic leukemia
   (C)   aplastic anemia
   (D)   hairy cell leukemia
   (E)   leukemoid reaction

207. The cause of the severe hemorrhage in acute promyelocytic leukemia is

   (A)   disseminated intravascular coagulation
   (B)   immune complex deposits on blood vessels
   (C)   thrombocytopenia
   (D)   thrombocytosis
   (E)   vascular damage from chemotherapy

A 60 year-old man had a 3 month history of increasing weight loss. He had hepato- and splenomegaly. His skin showed petechiae. His white blood cell count was 60,000/mm³. A photomicrograph of his peripheral blood smear is shown in Figure 3.1.

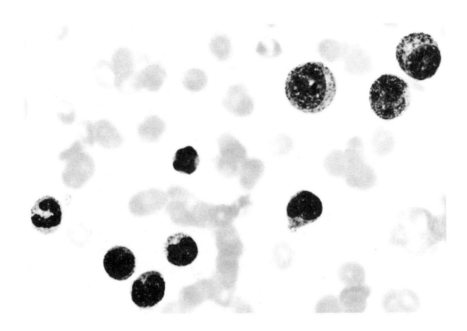

Figure 3.1

208. The likeliest diagnosis is

    (A)   acute myeloblastic leukemia
    (B)   acute promyelocytic leukemia
    (C)   chronic myelocytic leukemia
    (D)   hairy cell leukemia
    (E)   leukemoid reaction

209. Features of chronic myelocytic leukemia include all of the following **EXCEPT**:

    (A)   autoimmune hemolytic anemia
    (B)   conversion to acute leukemia (blast crisis)
    (C)   hyperviscosity of blood
    (D)   low alkaline phosphatase level in leukemic granulocytes
    (E)   Philadelphia chromosome in over 85 percent of cases

210. A 5 year-old child developed fever, hemorrhages, and repeated infections. Her white blood cell count was 50,000/mm³, and a blood smear showed immature white cells. A diagnosis of leukemia was made. The commonest form of leukemia in childhood is

  (A) acute myeloblastic leukemia
  (B) chronic myelocytic leukemia
  (C) acute lymphoblastic leukemia
  (D) chronic lymphocytic leukemia
  (E) hairy cell leukemia

211. A 60 year-old man gradually developed weakness and lymphadenopathy. His white blood count was 30,000/mm³ with predominantly small mature lymphocytes on peripheral and bone marrow smears. A diagnosis of chronic lymphocytic leukemia (CLL) was made. Characteristic features of CLL include all of the following **EXCEPT**:

  (A) autoimmune hemolytic anemia
  (B) conversion to acute leukemia (blast crisis)
  (C) hepatomegaly and splenomegaly
  (D) immunologically incompetent B lymphocytes
  (E) thrombocytopenia

212. Characteristic features of hairy cell leukemia include all of the following **EXCEPT**:

  (A) B lymphocyte origin in most cases
  (B) lymphocytes with filamentous cytoplasmic projections
  (C) splenectomy is often beneficial
  (D) tartrate resistant acid phosphatase in hairy cells
  (E) translocation from chromosome 17 to 15 in hairy cells

ANSWERS AND TUTORIAL ON ITEMS 204-212

The answers are: **204-A; 205-A; 206-B; 207-A; 208-C; 209-A; 210-C; 211-B; 212-E**.

In Item 204, the sudden onset with a severe infection, markedly elevated white cell count, and very immature myeloid cells (myeloblasts) in the peripheral blood are indicative of acute myeloblastic leukemia. Auer rods in the cytoplasm of myeloblasts are a distinctive feature in AML.

In Item 206, extensive hemorrhages are more characteristic of acute promyelocytic leukemia than other leukemias. The bleeding is mainly due to triggering of disseminated intravascular coagulation with subsequent hemorrhage.

In Item 208, the age of the patient, chronicity, splenic enlargement, very high white blood cell count, and mixture of mature and immature myeloid cells in the peripheral blood point to chronic myelocytic leukemia (CML). A blast crisis with conversion to acute myeloblastic (occasionally lymphoblastic) leukemia is a common cause of death. The low alkaline phosphatase in leukemic granulocytes is a useful indicator in distinguishing between leukemia and a leukemoid reaction. The Philadelphia chromosome (t 9q+; 22q-) is most typical of CML, but occurs in other forms of leukemia. The (t 15q+; 17q-) is found in acute promyelocytic leukemia; (t 14q+; 8q-) occurs in Burkitt's lymphoma.

In Item 210, acute lymphoblastic leukemia (ALL) is the characteristic leukemia of childhood; it has a second peak in older adults.

In Item 211, the age, chronicity, and large numbers of immunologically incompetent, mature, small B lymphocytes in the peripheral blood and bone marrow typify chronic lymphocytic leukemia (CLL). An autoimmune hemolytic anemia sometimes occurs in CLL. Liver and splenic enlargement are common, and there is an anemia and thrombocytopenia due to lymphocytic proliferation in the bone marrow, crowding out other cell elements. Blast crisis almost never occurs in CLL.

Leukemia is a malignant neoplastic proliferation of leukoblastic tissue. There is evidence that viruses, ionizing radiation, prolonged exposure to benzene, and genetic mutations are involved. Type C oncornaviruses cause leukemia in primates, and type C retrovirus (HTLV-I) has been isolated from human cases of T cell leukemia. Acute leukemia is common in children with trisomy 21. In over 85 percent of cases of chronic myelocytic leukemia, there is an abnormally small chromosome 22 with translocation on chromosome 9 (t 9q+; 22q-) (Philadelphia chromosome).

Acute myeloblastic (myelogenous) leukemia (AML) occurs at any age and is more common in males than females. Large infiltrates of bones, especially the skull, produce greenish masses known as chloromas. The peripheral blood shows a moderate elevation in the number of white cells, most of which are very immature granulocytic cells (myeloblasts and promyelocytes). Similar cells predominate in the bone marrow. The presence of eosinophilic rods (Auer bodies) within the cytoplasm distinguishes myelocytic from other types of immature cells. The leukemic cells crowd out erythroid precursors and megakaryocytes, so that anemia and hemorrhages are common. The neutrophilic cells in the blood are immature and ineffective against bacterial invasion. Untreated cases usually die within 6 months, death being the result of hemorrhage, frequently into the brain, or bacterial or mycotic infection. An increased incidence of AML has been noted in patients undergoing chemotherapy or radiotherapy.

Acute promyelocytic leukemia (APL) is characterized by more severe hemorrhagic phenomena than those of other acute leukemias. The patient may present with massive ecchymoses, hematuria, epistaxis, or menometrorrhagia. The hemorrhagic diathesis results from disseminated intravascular coagulation. In the bone marrow, more than 50 percent of cells are promyelocytes. About 40 percent of patients with APL have a chromosomal abnormality with translocation from the long arm of 17 to 15 (t 15q+; 17q-).

Chronic myelocytic leukemia (CML) develops gradually with fatigue, skin pallor and weight loss. It tends to occur after 50. In the peripheral blood and marrow, there is a mixture of immature and mature granulocytic cells. In CML, the white count may be extremely high ($>$ 2×10^5 WBC/mm^3). Organ infiltration by leukemic cells is common. The spleen may become very large, and there are lesser enlargements of the liver, kidneys, and lymph nodes. Hemorrhages, due to thrombocytopenia or thrombocytosis with formation of ineffective platelets, and anemia are frequent. Increased blood viscosity due to the large number of granulocytes may cause thrombosis and infarction, especially in the spleen. Average survival time is about 4 years. Death may be due to a "blast crisis" (conversion into acute leukemia) or infection. The latter may be bacterial or mycotic and often involves the lungs. The crisis is usually myeloblastic but may be lymphoblastic. In lymphoid blast crisis, the cells often have the Philadelphia chromosome.

Acute lymphoblastic leukemia (ALL) occurs mainly in children. T-cell markers are found in 25 percent of cases. In almost all other cases, the leukemic cells lack markers and are known as null cells. The cells of common non-T, non-B ALL appear to be primitive B cells. There is an abrupt onset with fever, weakness, hemorrhages, and infections. Lymphoblasts predominate in the peripheral blood and lymph nodes, and these cells infiltrate the bone marrow. The peripheral white count is usually $< 10^5/mm^3$. With chemotherapy, affected children may survive for several years.

Chronic lymphocytic leukemia (CLL) usually develops after 40 and is commoner in men than women. It is a disorder of B lymphocytes. The neoplastic cells consist of some lymphoblasts, but most resemble mature lymphocytes. Liver infiltration is typically more marked than in myelocytic leukemia, and the spleen is less enlarged in lymphocytic leukemia. Lymph node enlargement is pronounced. Hemorrhages, anemia, and infections may result from crowding out of megakaryocytes, erythroid cells, and granulocytes from the bone marrow. An autoimmune hemolytic anemia also occurs with CLL. About 60 percent of patients with CLL have hypogammaglobulinemia.

Hairy cell leukemia is rare and is characterized by splenomegaly, lymphadenopathy, and the presence of hairy cells in the peripheral blood, bone marrow, and spleen. These are cells resembling large lymphocytes which have fine, filamentous cytoplasmic projections and an eccentric, indented nucleus with lacy chromatin and prominent nucleolus. The origin of the hairy cell is a monoclonal B cell proliferation in most cases. Tartrate-resistant acid phosphatase is present in the cytoplasm of these cells. The course is chronic, and splenectomy produces a good response. A subtype of human T-cell leukemia virus (HTLV-II) has been found in the T-cell variant of hairy cell leukemia.

Items 213-223

213.   A 60 year-old man complained of bone pain, especially in his spine. X-rays revealed lytic lesions in the vertebrae and skull. He also had anemia and hypercalcemia. The likeliest diagnosis is

(A)   Burkitt's lymphoma
(B)   chronic lymphocytic lymphoma
(C)   heavy chain disease
(D)   multiple myeloma
(E)   Waldenström's macroglobulinemia

214. Characteristic findings in this man's disease include all of the following **EXCEPT**:

    (A) Bence-Jones proteinuria
    (B) decreased resistance to infection
    (C) infiltration of flat bones by plasma cells
    (D) macroglobulinemia
    (E) monoclonal gammopathy

215. Characteristic findings in Waldenström's macroglobulinemia include all of the following **EXCEPT**:

    (A) excessive production of immunoglobulin heavy chains
    (B) hemorrhages into skin and gums
    (C) hyperviscosity of blood
    (D) increased levels of IgM
    (E) plasmacytoid cells in lymph nodes and spleen

216. All of the following are usually disorders of B lymphocytes **EXCEPT**:

    (A) Burkitt's lymphoma
    (B) chronic lymphocytic leukemia
    (C) follicular (nodular) lymphoma
    (D) Hodgkin's disease
    (E) Waldenström's macroglobulinemia

217. An association with an increased incidence of lymphomas has been found with all of the following **EXCEPT**:

    (A) autoimmune disorders
    (B) chromosome abnormalities
    (C) cigarette smoking
    (D) immune deficiencies
    (E) viruses

218. A 40 year-old man presented with weight loss and painless lymphadenopathy. A node biopsy showed proliferation of germinal centers in the cortex and medulla. The enlarged centers consisted of poorly differentiated lymphocytes. The likeliest diagnosis is

    (A) acute lymphadenitis
    (B) Burkitt's lymphoma
    (C) diffuse poorly differentiated lymphocytic lymphoma
    (D) follicular (nodular) lymphocytic lymphoma
    (E) lymphocyte predominance Hodgkin's disease

219. Characteristic findings in Burkitt's lymphoma include all of the following **EXCEPT**:

  (A)   Epstein-Barr virus is causally implicated
  (B)   lymph nodes are not commonly involved
  (C)   osteolytic lesions in jaw bones are frequent
  (D)   translocation from chromosome 8 to 14 is common
  (E)   the tumor is unresponsive to chemotherapy

A 25 year-old woman had recurrent low grade fever and cervical lymphadenopathy. Photomicrographs of a lymph node biopsy are in Figure 3.2.

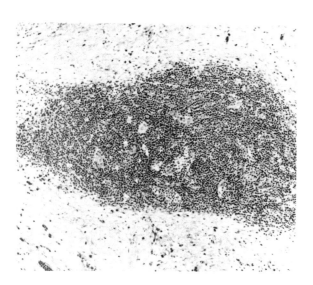 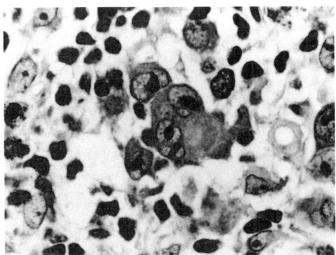

Figure 3.2

220. The likeliest diagnosis is

  (A)   Burkitt's lymphoma
  (B)   chronic lymphadenitis
  (C)   histiocytic lymphoma
  (D)   Hodgkin's disease
  (E)   nodular lymphoma

221. All of the following statements are true concerning Hodgkin's disease **EXCEPT**:

   (A)   Burkitt's lymphoma is a variant occurring in Africa
   (B)   leukemia and other malignancies have appeared in patients successfully treated for Hodgkin's disease
   (C)   lymph nodes and spleen are commonly involved
   (D)   nodular sclerosis type is the commonest form
   (E)   Reed-Sternberg cells are the most important diagnostic feature

222. The patient in Item 220 would most likely have which of the following types of Hodgkin's disease?

   (A)   lymphocyte depletion
   (B)   lymphocyte predominance
   (C)   mixed cellularity
   (D)   nodular sclerosis

223. The patient in Item 220 was found to have involvement of the cervical and mediastinal lymph nodes and spleen. The extent of the disease was

   (A)   Stage I A
   (B)   Stage II B
   (C)   Stage III A
   (D)   Stage III B
   (E)   Stage IV B

ANSWERS AND TUTORIAL ON ITEMS 213-223

The answers are: **213-D; 214-D; 215-A; 216-D; 217-C; 218-D; 219-E; 220-D; 221-A; 222-D; 223-D**.

> In Item 213, the age, bone pain, lytic lesions in flat bones, hypercalcemia, and anemia are indicative of multiple myeloma (MM). Macroglobulinemia is not typical of MM.
>
> Lymphomas occur in increased incidence in autoimmune disorders such as rheumatoid arthritis and lupus erythematosus; chromosome defects, such as t 18q+; 14q- in follicular lymphoma; both congenital and acquired immunodeficiencies, such as AIDS; and exposure to certain viruses, such as Epstein-Barr in Burkitt's lymphoma.
>
> In Item 218, the overgrowth of poorly differentiated lymphocytes throughout the lymph nodes in a pattern mimicking germinal centers is typical of nodular lymphoma.
>
> In Item 220, the age, sex, recurrent fever and lymphadenopathy, sclerosis, lacunar cells, the Reed-Sternberg cell, and eosinophils are characteristic of the nodular sclerosis type of Hodgkin's disease. Involvement of lymph nodes and spleen (on both sides of the diaphragm) and the presence of symptoms would place this case in Stage III B.

Plasma cell dyscrasias are characterized by malignant neoplastic or other abnormal proliferation of plasma cells and include multiple (plasma cell) myeloma; solitary myeloma; soft tissue plasmacytoma; plasma cell leukemia; and reactive plasma cell proliferation. These all arise in B lymphocytes. Patients with plasma cell neoplasms have high levels of immunoglobulin. Each produces a specific type which stays constant (monoclonal gammopathy). This appears as a single, well-defined spike on electrophoresis (myeloma or M-protein). The globulin is usually of the IgG type. Myeloma globulins lack receptor sites and so have no antibody activity. Over half of patients with plasma cell myeloma produce Bence-Jones protein, which consists of 2 immunoglobulin light chains linked by a disulfide bond. This protein is small enough to appear in the urine.

In multiple myeloma, the vertebrae, ribs, and skull are most often involved by an overgrowth of plasma cells. Production of an osteoclast activating factor produces erosion of cortical bone and hypercalcemia. Soft tissue plasmacytoma occurs most often in the upper respiratory tract or mouth. In the kidneys, Bence-Jones protein casts are frequently found in the tubules. Multinucleated foreign body giant cell reaction occurs among the tubular lining cells. Amyloidosis involving the myocardium and other organs develops in about 10 percent of cases of plasma cell dyscrasia.

Waldenström's macroglobulinemia is characterized by production of strikingly increased levels of IgM. It is a disorder of B lymphocytes and occurs most commonly in men 50-70 years old. Cardiac failure may result from increased viscosity of the blood. About 10 percent of the patients have Bence-Jones protein in the urine. There are diffuse infiltrates of lymphoid plasmacytes in the bone marrow, lymph nodes, and spleen. The lymphoid plasmacyte has an eccentric ovoid nucleus and ample cytoplasm, sometimes with a clear zone about the nucleus. Eosinophilic, PAS positive Dutcher bodies, consisting of IgM, may be present in its cytoplasm and nucleus.

Lymphomas are malignant neoplasms of lymphoid cells. They are usually primary in lymph nodes but occasionally begin in the intestine, spleen, or other organs. Lymphomas most often arise in B lymphocytes. Involved lymph nodes are enlarged and pinkish gray. They may be discrete or matted. In follicular (nodular) lymphoma, there is an increase in the number and size of lymph follicles. These usually consist of small, poorly differentiated lymphocytes. Lymphomas of diffuse types show a monotonous pattern of cells throughout the involved nodes and invading the perinodal tissue. Well differentiated lymphocytic lymphomas consist of sheets of small, mature-appearing lymphocytes. Poorly differentiated lymphocytic lymphomas are made up of large, poorly differentiated lymphocytes. Histiocytic lymphomas are formed by transformed lymphocytes (only about 1 percent of "histiocytic" lymphomas are truly of histiocytic origin). Undifferentiated lymphomas consist of large, lymphoblastic cells and scattered pale histiocytes with abundant cytoplasm containing phagocytized material.

Burkitt's lymphoma occurs in children endemically across central Africa and sporadically elsewhere. Many patients have a chromosomal translocation from the long arm of 8 to 14 (t 8q-; 14q+). The neoplasm develops most commonly in the jaws, abdomen, and retroperitoneal soft tissues. There may be little or no lymph node involvement. The jaw lesion is an osteolytic one in the maxilla or mandible. In untreated cases, death occurs within a few weeks or months. Apparent cures have been achieved by the administration of cyclophosphamide.

Hodgkin's disease (HD) is a malignant neoplasm mainly involving lymph nodes. The cause is unknown. The exfoliant Agent Orange has been implicated as a cause of both HD and non-Hodgkin's lymphomas. Many patients are unable to develop a normal delayed hypersensitivity reaction, so that defective immune surveillance may be involved in the pathogenesis of Hodgkin's disease. The indispensable feature for the diagnosis of HD is the Reed-Sternberg (R-S) cell. This is a large cell with multiple nuclei or a multilobed nucleus. The latter has a prominent, often eosinophilic nucleolus. Evidence indicates that the R-S cell arises from an interdigitating reticular cell. HD has been classified into 4 types. The lymphocyte predominance type has the best prognosis. The involved nodes show only a few R-S cells and eosinophils within uniform sheets or nodules of lymphocytes. In the nodular sclerosis form, there are nodules consisting of R-S cells, mononuclear R-S cells in spaces (lacunar cells), eosinophils, and lymphocytes separated by dense fibrous bands. The mixed cellularity type shows a heterogenous mixture of R-S and atypical histiocytes, eosinophils, neutrophils, and lymphocytes and varying amounts of fibrous tissue. The lymphocyte depletion type has a poor prognosis. Involved nodes consist almost entirely of Reed-Sternberg cells and atypical histiocytes. HD involves lymph nodes, such as the cervical, mediastinal, mesenteric, and retroperitoneal groups, and spleen mainly. Infiltration of organs such as the liver, lungs, and kidneys occurs in the mixed cell and lymphocytic depletion forms. Acute non-lymphocytic leukemia and other second malignant neoplasms have developed in a number of cases of HD and non-Hodgkin's lymphoma treated with chemotherapy and/or radiotherapy.

Lymphomas and Hodgkin's disease are staged as: (1) Stage I - disease limited to one anatomic region; (2) Stage II - disease involving 2 or 3 regions on same side of diaphragm; (3) Stage III - disease on both sides of diaphragm but limited to lymph nodes, spleen, and Waldeyer's ring (tonsils and adenoids); and (4) Stage IV - disease involving visceral organs in addition to lymph nodes, spleen, and oropharyngeal lymphoid tissue. Any stage is subclassified as A if the patient has no systemic manifestation, or B if he or she has signs and symptoms such as fever and itching.

Items 224-229

224.   A 30 year-old woman developed purpura in her skin and hematuria. She had been healthy and used no drugs. Her platelet count was 40,000/mm³, red cell count 4.5 million/mm³, and white cell count 8000/mm³. The likeliest presumptive diagnosis is

        (A)   disseminated intravascular coagulation
        (B)   primary (idiopathic) thrombocytopenic purpura
        (C)   secondary thrombocytopenic purpura
        (D)   thrombotic thrombocytopenic purpura
        (E)   aplastic anemia

225. Features of this woman's disease include all of the following **EXCEPT**:

   (A) anti-platelet antibodies are present
   (B) bleeding time is prolonged
   (C) coagulation time is usually normal
   (D) large hemorrhages occur in the skin and GI tract
   (E) splenomegaly is common

226. Secondary thrombocytopenic purpura may occur in all of the following **EXCEPT**:

   (A) aplastic anemia
   (B) leukemias
   (C) metastatic carcinoma to bones
   (D) patients using quinidine
   (E) von Willebrand's disease

227. A young boy had excessive bleeding from minor wounds and even spontaneously. He was found to have a severe deficiency of coagulation factor VIII. Factor IX levels were normal, as was platelet adhesiveness. The likeliest diagnosis is

   (A) Christmas disease
   (B) hemophilia
   (C) Stuart factor deficiency
   (D) von Willebrand's disease

228. All of the following are true concerning hemophilia **EXCEPT**:

   (A) antihemophilic globulin is present in normal amounts in some patients
   (B) bleeding time is normal
   (C) clot retraction does not occur
   (D) coagulation time is prolonged
   (E) hemarthroses are common

229. A 30 year-old woman with an acute illness developed hemorrhages into the skin as well as signs of multiple thromboses. Disseminated intravascular coagulation (DIC) was diagnosed. DIC may be triggered by all of the following **EXCEPT**:

   (A) amniotic fluid embolism
   (B) gram-negative septicemia
   (C) premature separation of placenta
   (D) rattlesnake venom
   (E) streptokinase

ANSWERS AND TUTORIAL ON ITEMS 224-229

The answers are: **224-B; 225-D; 226-E; 227-B; 228-C; 229-E**. Primary (idiopathic) thrombocytopenic purpura (ITP) is an autoimmune disease. Anti-platelet antibodies are found as IgG directed against platelet-associated antigen. The spleen destroys platelets coated by auto-antibodies, and by producing these antibodies. Splenectomy leads to remission or cure in most cases. The platelet count is commonly reduced to below 50,000/mm^3. The bleeding time is prolonged, and the coagulation time is normal unless the platelets are reduced to an extremely low level. Clot retraction does not occur. Platelet survival time is strikingly reduced.

In ITP small hemorrhages occur in the skin, brain, and respiratory, gastrointestinal, and genitourinary mucosa. The spleen is enlarged. The germinal centers are large and active. In the bone marrow, the number of megakaryocytes is usually increased, but many of them are immature forms.

Secondary thrombocytopenic purpura is caused by a number of therapeutic agents. Drugs may produce thrombocytopenia by direct depression of the production of platelets in the bone marrow or by decreasing the life span of platelets through the development of anti-platelet antibodies. Drugs which cause thrombocytopenia include quinidine, heparin, and cancer chemotherapeutic agents. Thrombocytopenic purpura also occurs in the leukemias, metastatic carcinoma in bone marrow, aplastic anemia, benzene poisoning, radiation therapy, or chronic infection. In all of these, platelet formation is interfered with by direct invasion of the bone marrow or by marrow hypoplasia caused by the action of toxins.

Hemophilia is inherited as a recessive sex-linked characteristic and occurs almost always in males. Most patients have very low levels of coagulation factor VIII (antihemophilic globulin, AHG). In about 10 percent of cases, even though the amount of AHG is normal, a functionally defective form is found. In hemophilia, the coagulation time is prolonged, and the bleeding time is normal. Clot retraction is prompt, once coagulation occurs. In hemophilia, there is excessive and sometimes fatal bleeding from minor wounds as well as spontaneous hemorrhages in the gums, gastrointestinal tract, and joints. Hemarthroses occur in about half the cases, the knees, ankles, and elbows being most frequently involved.

Disseminated intravascular coagulation (DIC) is characterized by bleeding resulting from the using up of coagulation factors by excessive intravascular clotting. It develops in the human equivalent of the Shwartzman phenomenon, which occurs in septicemia due to gram-negative bacteria. Widespread intracapillary fibrin thrombosis is triggered by activation of Hageman factor and the release of thromboplastin. The latter also initiates disseminated intravascular clotting in premature placental separation and amniotic fluid embolism. In DIC, various hemorrhagic phenomena occur.

230. Cells which play a primary role in immune reactions include all of the following **EXCEPT**:

    (A) eosinophils
    (B) lymphocytes
    (C) macrophages
    (D) mast cells
    (E) neutrophils

231. A 20 year-old man with a history of hypersensitivity to bee venom was stung. He had a severe reaction with swelling and redness around the sting site. Important factors which play a role in such a reaction include all of the following **EXCEPT**:

    (A) B-lymphocytes
    (B) eosinophils
    (C) histamine
    (D) IgE
    (E) mast cells

232. Within minutes after restoring circulation in a transplanted kidney, the organ became pale and began to show foci of necrosis. In such hyperacute rejection the dominant pathologic change is

    (A) acute necrotizing vasculitis
    (B) acute inflammation with abscess formation
    (C) an Arthus reaction
    (D) infiltration of cytotoxic T-lymphocytes
    (E) granulomatous inflammation

233. The type of hypersensitivity reaction in hyperacute rejection is

    (A) Type I (immediate)
    (B) Type II (antibody dependent)
    (C) Type III (immune complex)
    (D) Type IV (cell-mediated)

234. All of the following are important factors which play a role in antibody dependent hypersensitivity **EXCEPT**:

(A) antigen on cell surfaces
(B) complement
(C) eosinophils
(D) IgG
(E) natural killer cells

235. After performing satisfactorily for a month, a transplanted kidney began to show signs of rejection. A biopsy showed an interstitial infiltrate of T-lymphocytes and macrophages. There was only slight vasculitis. The type of hypersensitivity reaction in this acute rejection is

(A) Type I (immediate)
(B) Type II (antibody dependent)
(C) Type III (immune complex)
(D) Type IV (cell-mediated)

In Items 236-245, match the disorder with the type of immune mechanism which is associated with it.

(A) Type I (immediate hypersensitivity)
(B) Type II (antibody dependent hypersensitivity)
(C) Type III (immune complex hypersensitivity)
(D) Type IV (cell-mediated hypersensitivity)

236. asthma

237. autoimmune hemolytic anemia

238. contact dermatitis to poison ivy

239. erythroblastosis fetalis

240. Goodpasture's syndrome

241. hay fever

242. lupus erythematosus

243. polyarteritis nodosa

244. post-streptococcal glomerulonephritis

245. urticaria

ANSWERS AND TUTORIAL ON ITEMS 230-245

The answers are: 230-E; 231-A; 232-A; 233-B; 234-C; 235-D; 236-A; 237-B; 238-D; 239-B; 240-B; 241-A; 242-C; 243-C; 244-C; 245-A.

Insect stings invoke a Type I (immediate hypersensitivity reaction) in which binding of IgE to mast cells leads to release of histamine, and eosinophil chemotactic factor attracts eosinophils. Lymphocytes play no role in this reaction.

In Item 232, hyperacute rejection is caused by preexisting circulating antibodies to antigens in the graft. Such rejection is an example of a Type II reaction and is characterized by an acute necrotizing vasculitis. Eosinophils play no role in hyperacute rejection.

In Item 235, development of a cell-mediated hypersensitivity reaction is mainly responsible for acute rejection, although circulating antibodies to tissue antigens may play a role by causing a vasculitis.

In Items 236-245, asthma, hay fever, and urticaria are due to Type I hypersensitivity; autoimmune hemolytic anemia, erythroblastosis fetalis, and Goodpasture's syndrome, to Type II; lupus erythematosus, polyarteritis nodosa, and post-streptococcal glomerulonephritis, Type III; and contact dermatitis, Type IV.

Hypersensitivity (allergy) is a phenomenon in which an immunologic response is the cause of reactions damaging to body cells. Antigens producing such harmful effects are allergens. The types of allergic reaction are: Type I, immediate hypersensitivity; Type II, antibody dependent hypersensitivity; Type III, immune complex hypersensitivity; and Type IV, cell-mediated hypersensitivity.

Type I immediate hypersensitivity reaction is usually a result of an initial parenteral sensitization followed some time later by a second exposure to the sensitizing antigen. It is due to the binding of IgE to sensitized mast cells. The chemical mediators of these reactions are histamine, eosinophil chemotactic factor of anaphylaxis (ECF-A), and slow reacting substance of anaphylaxis (SRS-A). Eosinophils accumulate at the site of reaction. IgE mediated hypersensitivities such as hay fever, asthma, and urticaria, represent mild forms of anaphylaxis.

Type II antibody dependent hypersensitivity is due to circulating antibodies against antigens present on cells or other tissue elements. Cell or tissue injury may be due to attachment of antibodies to antigens and activation of complement or the action of natural killer cells. Complement activation may lead to damage to erythrocyte membranes by the membrane attack complex (C'56789).

Soluble antigen-antibody (immune) complexes are formed in the presence of antigen excess. When complexes of optimal size develop, a soluble immune complex (Type III) reaction occurs. The soluble complexes fix complement, and C'5a is chemotactic for neutrophils. Proteolytic enzymes released from lysosomes of neutrophils cause tissue damage locally, especially to vascular endothelium and basement membranes. Diseases due to the development of a soluble immune complex reaction include serum sickness, polyarteritis nodosa, disseminated lupus erythematosus, and post-streptococcal glomerulonephritis. The Arthus phenomenon is also caused by it.

Type IV cell-mediated (delayed) hypersensitivity is important in immune surveillance, as in acute homograft rejection and the elimination of mutant cells; in resistance to infections

94

by intracellular parasites, such as <u>Mycobacterium tuberculosis</u>, rickettsiae, and viruses; and in some autoimmune diseases. Grossly an erythematous, indurated focus appears at the reaction site. Microscopically the infiltrating cells are mainly T-lymphocytes and macrophages. The triggering event in cell-mediated hypersensitivity is the interaction of receptors on the T-lymphocyte surface with antigen. Some sensitized lymphocytes are cytotoxic. Sensitized T-lymphocytes liberate lymphokines. Macrophages accumulate and their phagocytosis is enhanced. Macrophages also process antigen for interaction with T-lymphocytes. Tissue necrosis in cell-mediated hypersensitivity is nonselective and involves all cell elements. It is due to release of lymphotoxin, the effects of cytotoxic T cells, and release of lysosomal enzymes from macrophages.

Items 246-262

In Items 246-251, match the antigen with the organ specific autoimmune disease in which it is a principal target.

      (A)   Addison's disease
      (B)   Goodpasture's syndrome
      (C)   Graves' disease (primary hyperthyroidism)
      (D)   idiopathic thrombocytopenic purpura
      (E)   juvenile diabetes mellitus
      (F)   lymphocytic (Hashimoto's) thyroiditis
      (G)   myasthenia gravis
      (H)   pernicious anemia

246.   acetylcholine receptor

247.   gastric parietal cells

248.   glomerular and lung basement membranes

249.   microsomal antigen

250.   pancreatic islet cells

251.   thyroid stimulating hormone (TSH) receptor

A 30 year-old man developed fever, hypertension, abdominal pain, skin lesions, joint swelling, and proteinuria. A photomicrograph of a biopsy of one of the lesions is shown in Figure 3.3.

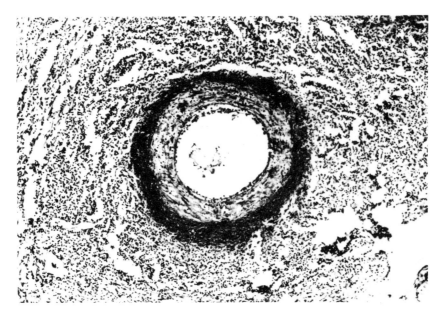

Figure 3.3

252. The likeliest diagnosis is

(A) amyloidosis
(B) lupus erythematosus
(C) polyarteritis nodosa
(D) rheumatoid arthritis
(E) systemic sclerosis

253. A 30 year-old woman complained of joint pains and swelling. She had an erythematous rash acoss the nose and cheeks, proteinuria, and pancytopenia. The likeliest diagnosis is

(A) dermatomyositis
(B) disseminated lupus erythematosus (DLE)
(C) polyarteritis nodosa
(D) rheumatoid arthritis
(E) systemic sclerosis

254. Of the following autoantibodies the one which is most characteristic of disseminated lupus erythematosus is

   (A) anti DNA
   (B) antierythrocyte
   (C) antimitochondrial
   (D) antinucleoprotein
   (E) antithyroglobulin

In Items 255-261, match the item with the disease with which each is most closely associated.

   (A) amyloidosis
   (B) dermatomyositis
   (C) disseminated lupus erythematosus
   (D) polyarteritis nodosa
   (E) progressive systemic sclerosis (scleroderma)

255. collagenous thickening of dermis

256. fibrinoid necrosis of medium-sized arteries

257. hematoxylin bodies

258. immunoglobulin light chain deposition in glomeruli

259. increased incidence of malignant neoplasms

260. soluble immune complex deposits in glomeruli

261. sterile vegetations on heart valves

262. Amyloid deposits are associated with all of the following **EXCEPT**:

   (A) Alzheimer's disease
   (B) chronic osteomyelitis
   (C) multiple myeloma
   (D) syphilis
   (E) tuberculosis of lungs

ANSWERS AND TUTORIAL ON ITEMS 246-262

The answers are: **246-G; 247-H; 248-B; 249-F; 250-E; 251-C; 252-C; 253-B; 254-A; 255-E; 256-D; 257-C; 258-A; 259-B; 260-C; 261-C; 262-D**.

Items 246 to 251 are targets in organ specific autoimmune disease. Antiacetylcholine receptor antibodies, acting at the myoneural junction, cause the muscle weakness in myasthenia gravis. In pernicious anemia an atrophic gastritis and failure to produce intrinsic factor necessary for vitamin B_{12} absorption is caused by antiparietal cell antibodies. Anti-glomerular and -lung basement membrane antibodies cause pulmonary hemorrhages and glomerulonephritis in Goodpasture's syndrome. Anti-microsomal (and antithyroglobulin) antibodies are responsible for the development of lymphocytic thyroiditis. In juvenile diabetes islet ß-cells are destroyed by antibodies against them. In Graves' disease anti-TSH receptor antibodies simulate TSH and cause excessive thyroid hormone production.

In Item 252, the photomicrograph shows fibrinoid necrosis and neutrophilic infiltration in and around the wall of a small artery. These findings are characteristic of polyarteritis nodosa.

In Item 253, the age, sex, butterfly rash, renal involvement, and low blood cell counts all point to lupus erythematosus. Of the multitude of autoantibodies in DLE, anti DNA and the formation and deposition of DNA-anti DNA complexes are most important.

In Items 255 to 261 collagenous dermal thickening is typical of scleroderma; fibrinoid vascular necrosis of polyarteritis; hematoxylin bodies (complexes of nucleoprotein-antinucleoprotein) of DLE; an increased incidence of cancer of dermatomyositis; and glomerular immune complex deposits and valvular vegetations of DLE.

In Item 262 amyloids are deposited in senile plaques and small arteries in the brain in Alzheimer's disease, in the liver, spleen and kidneys in prolonged infections, such as osteomyelitis and tuberculosis, and as Ig light chains in multiple myeloma. Deposits are not found in syphilis.

Autoimmune disease is a hypersensitivity to self-antigen. Autoimmunity itself is normal. Anti-idiotype antibodies and T-suppressor cells recognize and neutralize self antibodies and antiself lymphocytes. Autoimmune disease results from uncontrolled proliferation of a clone of T-helper lymphocytes directed against self-antigens on non-lymphoid cells. The production of such a clone may be due to genetic susceptibility, an environmental trigger such as a virus, or failure of tolerance and suppressor mechanisms.

Polyarteritis (periarteritis) nodosa is a soluble immune complex disease with localization of antigen-antibody complexes on blood vessel walls. In about half of the cases immune complexes containing hepatitis B antigen are found on affected tissues.

Multiple small and medium-sized arteries are usually affected. Arterioles, venules, and capillaries (including the glomerular tufts) may also be involved. In acute cases there is smudgy fibrinoid necrosis of the walls of the vessels, obliterating evidence of the normal muscular layers, and eosinophils and neutrophils are found throughout all portions of the vessel walls including the adventitia. In more chronic cases, there is often a foreign body reaction in the vessel walls.

Disseminated lupus erythematosus (DLE) is an autoimmune type of soluble immune complex disease in which DNA-anti DNA complexes are formed. The disorder occurs most commonly in women 18 to 35 years of age. Besides anti DNA antibodies, antinucleoprotein, antinucleolar, antimitochondrial, antierythrocyte, anti-T-lymphocyte, antithrombin, antithyroglobulin and many other autoantibodies have been found in patients with DLE. The cause is unknown. Hereditary susceptibility, viruses, and an immune defect have been implicated. Cell-mediated immunity is defective in DLE. A disease identical with or very similar to DLE has developed in persons taking hydralazine and procainamide. Pathologic changes may involve almost any organ. The characteristic lesion is fibrinoid necrosis of collagen and small arteries. Immunoglobulin, complement, and fibrinogen are demonstrated by immunofluorescence in vascular lesions. The vasculitis is caused by a soluble immune complex reaction. The kidneys may be large and pale on gross examination. Microscopically the glomerular lesions are pleomorphic; they may be focal, membranous, or mesangial. The changes are mainly due to subendothelial deposition of immune complexes. The heart often shows no changes grossly; however, in some cases small sterile fibrinous masses are seen along the line of closure of the valve cusps and on the endocardium of the left atrium (nonbacterial endocarditis of Libman and Sacks). Microscopically hematoxylin bodies may be seen beneath the atrial endocardium and elsewhere. These bodies represent complexes of nucleoprotein and antinucleoprotein antibodies. Skin changes include fibrinoid changes in the collagen just beneath the epidermis and vacuoles, in the basal layer of epidermis.

Amyloidosis is the accumulation of amyloids in various body tissues. Amyloids are complex protein substances containing glycosaminoglycans. In the primary type and amyloidosis associated with plasma cell myeloma the amyloid consists of immunoglobulin light chains and probably represents abnormal Ig production. This amyloid is designated AL protein. Amyloid secondary to inflammatory processes is AA protein.

Primary amyloidosis is a rare disease having no demonstrable cause. The amyloid deposits occur in the tongue, skin, heart, gastrointestinal tract, and occasionally in and about the large joints more or less diffusely. Secondary amyloidosis is usually the late result of a long-continued inflammatory process involving bones, joints, or lungs, especially tuberculosis. Amyloidosis occurs in about 15 percent of cases of plasma cell myeloma. There is a heredofamilial form of amyloidosis. Isolated organ amyloidosis occurs with aging and in medullary carcinoma of the thyroid gland. Amyloid is present in senile plaques and small subarachnoid artery walls in Alzheimer's disease.

Items 263-267

263. All of the following are characteristic of Bruton's agammaglobulinemia **EXCEPT**:

   (A)   failure of pre B-lymphocytes to mature
   (B)   absence of follicles in lymph nodes and spleen
   (C)   development of leukemia
   (D)   recurrent pyogenic bacterial infections
   (E)   X-linked inheritance

264. All of the following are characteristic of DiGeorge's syndrome **EXCEPT**:

   (A)   hypoparathyroidism
   (B)   hypoplasia of T-dependent areas in lymph nodes
   (C)   inheritance as autosomal recessive
   (D)   recurrent viral and fungal infections
   (E)   absent thymus

265. An acquired immunodeficiency may occur in all of the following **EXCEPT**:

   (A)   adrenocorticosteroid therapy
   (B)   chronic lymphatic leukemia
   (C)   multiple myeloma
   (D)   progressive systemic sclerosis
   (E)   sarcoidosis

266. All of the following are immunodeficiency disorders **EXCEPT**:

   (A)   AIDS
   (B)   ataxia-telangiectasia
   (C)   chronic granulomatous disease
   (D)   Swiss type combined disease
   (E)   Wiskott-Aldrich syndrome

267. A striking increase in the incidence of malignant neoplasms occurs in patients with

   (A)   atopic disorders
   (B)   disseminated lupus erythematosus
   (C)   immune deficiency disorders
   (D)   scleroderma
   (E)   tuberculosis

ANSWERS AND TUTORIAL ON ITEMS 263-267

The answers are: **263-C; 264-C; 265-D; 266-C; 267-C**.

> There is no tendency to develop leukemia in Bruton's agammaglobulinemia. DiGeorge's syndrome is due to a developmental defect and is not inherited. Chronic granulomatous disease is due to an enzyme deficiency in neutrophils which leads to a failure to produce H_2O_2 and is a disorder of the inflammatory response. A markedly increased incidence of cancer is found in both congenital and acquired immunodeficiencies.

Infantile agammaglobulinemia (Bruton's disease) is an X-linked recessive disorder in which pre B-lymphocytes fail to mature so there is a deficiency of B-lymphocytes and thus plasma cells and immunoglobulins. The lymph nodes and spleen lack follicles. The humoral immune system is defective. Infections due to pyogenic bacteria are common.

Thymic aplasia (DiGeorge's syndrome) is due to failure of formation of the 3rd and 4th pharyngeal pouches. It is characterized by absence of the thymus and parathyroid glands. Lymph nodes show depletion in the T-dependent subcortical regions. The affected child has a deficient cell-mediated immune response. Immune globulins are normal or somewhat decreased. Viral and fungal infections are common, as is tetany from the parathyroid deficiency. Death usually occurs in early life.

An acquired immune defect in the form of hypo-γ-globulinemia may occur in diseases such as chronic lymphatic leukemia or lymphomas. It also occurs in plasma cell myeloma, in which abnormal immunoglobulin ineffective as antibody is formed; and in disorders characterized by excess loss or breakdown of plasma proteins, such as the nephrotic syndrome, extensive desquamative skin diseases, or protein-losing enteropathies. An acquired defect in cell-mediated immune response occurs in Hodgkin's disease and sarcoidosis.

Acquired immune deficiency syndrome is discussed with the Infectious Diseases.

Patients with either inherited, acquired, or induced forms of immune deficiencies, as well as those with autoimmune disease show an increased incidence of lymphoma and other forms of malignant neoplasia. This may be due to inadequacy of immune surveillance over the emergence of forbidden clones or the expression of viral oncogenes in malignant cells.

CHAPTER IV

RESPIRATORY PATHOLOGY

268. A middle aged homeless alcoholic was brought to the emergency room with chills, fever, dyspnea, cough, and rusty sputum. There was dullness over the right lower lobe. The likeliest diagnosis is

  (A)   bronchopneumonia
  (B)   lobar pneumonia
  (C)   mycoplasma pneumonia
  (D)   tuberculous pneumonia
  (E)   viral pneumonia

In Items 269-271, match each item with the type of pneumonia of which it is most descriptive microscopically.

  (A)   bronchopneumonia
  (B)   legionella pneumonia
  (C)   lobar pneumonia
  (D)   mycoplasma and viral pneumonia
  (E)   tuberculous pneumonia

269. hyaline membranes lining alveoli with mononuclear leukocytic infiltration of alveolar septa

270. patchy infiltration of alveolar spaces with neutrophils, especially around bronchioles

271. uniform infiltration of alveolar spaces with neutrophils and fibrin

272. Usual complications of pneumococcal lobar pneumonia include all of the following **EXCEPT**:

  (A)   empyema
  (B)   fibrinous pericarditis
  (C)   fibrinous pleuritis
  (D)   lung abscess
  (E)   organization

273. Bronchopneumonia is usually secondary to all of the following **EXCEPT**:

    (A)   aspiration into lungs
    (B)   congestion and edema of lungs
    (C)   influenzal pneumonia
    (D)   lipid pneumonia
    (E)   sarcoidosis of lungs

An 18 year-old male, with a history of malabsorption and steatorrhea since infancy, died after having chronic productive cough, hemoptysis, and recurrent pulmonary infections for several years. A photograph of a lung at autopsy is shown in Figure 4.1.

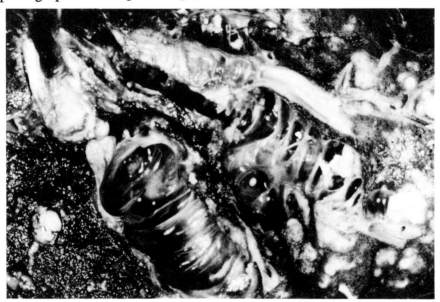

Figure 4.1

274. The likeliest diagnosis is

    (A)   bronchiectasis
    (B)   bronchopneumonia
    (C)   chronic pneumonitis
    (D)   lung abscess
    (E)   tuberculosis

275. The disease diagnosed in Item 274 may be secondary to all of the following **EXCEPT**:

   (A)   asthma
   (B)   bronchial obstruction due to carcinoma
   (C)   bronchial obstruction due to foreign body
   (D)   mucoviscidosis
   (E)   pertussis

276. A 40 year-old man developed fever and a cough with copious foul smelling sputum. A chest film showed a 5 cm. density with a fluid level in the right lower lobe. A lung abscess was diagnosed. Lung abscess may be secondary to all of the following **EXCEPT**:

   (A)   aspiration of oropharyngeal contents
   (B)   bronchial obstruction due to foreign body
   (C)   bronchiectasis
   (D)   organized pneumonia
   (E)   septic pulmonary embolism

277. Complications of chronic lung abscess include all of the following **EXCEPT**:

   (A)   brain abscess
   (B)   bronchopleural fistula
   (C)   empyema
   (D)   honeycomb lung
   (E)   secondary amyloidosis

ANSWERS AND TUTORIAL ON ITEMS 268-277

The answers are: **268-B; 269-D; 270-A; 271-C; 272-D; 273-E; 274-A; 275-A; 276-D; 277-D**.

In Item 268, the personal history and clinical findings all indicate the presence of a pneumonia. Involvement of a lobe on percussion points to lobar pneumonia. This is characterized by a uniform neutrophilic infiltration and fibrin within alveolar spaces. Lung abscess is not a usual complication of lobar pneumonia, although it does occur in some cases due to type 3 pneumococci and Klebsiella pneumoniae. Bronchopneumonia is usually secondary to some other pulmonary disorder. The intra-alveolar neutrophilic infiltrate is patchy and lobular rather than lobar (except in confluent bronchopneumonia). An interstitial leukocytic infiltrate with fibrinous membranes lining alveolar walls occurs in mycoplasma and viral pneumonias. Legionella pneumonia is variable in appearance from patchy to lobar in extent. Tuberculous pneumonia shows widespread caseation with neutrophils and few well-formed granulomata.

In Item 274, the young man had cystic fibrosis in which there are thick secretions from exocrine glands, including the bronchial mucous glands. Ropy mucus causes bronchial obstruction with infection and damage to bronchial walls leading to permanent dilatation (bronchiectasis). Other causes of bronchial obstruction and whooping cough may also lead to bronchiectasis.

In Item 276, lung abscess may develop from bacteria introduced into lungs by inhalation, hematogenously, or during chest trauma. Causative organisms may invade pulmonary veins and localize in the brain. They may produce a fistula into the pleural space or a loculated purulent exudate may develop there (empyema). Amyloidosis of the liver, spleen, and kidneys may complicate long standing lung abscess. Honeycomb lung is an end-stage condition not related to abscess.

Lobar pneumonia is almost always due to the pneumococcus, <u>Streptococcus</u> <u>pneumoniae</u>. About 5 percent of cases is caused by <u>Klebsiella</u> <u>pneumoniae</u>. Many individuals are carriers of pneumococci, and other factors besides the presence of the organisms appear to be necessary for the development of clinical disease. Among these are exposure to cold or dampness. Pneumonia is more common in debilitated persons and chronic alcoholics than in healthy individuals.

Red hepatization is the typical picture during the first three days of the disease. In this stage, the affected lobe is red, consolidated, and heavy. Microscopically the lung shows an intense hyperemia. The alveolar exudate consists of large numbers of red cells and neutrophils. Gray hepatization is the characteristic stage from the fourth to the eighth day in the typical course of untreated pneumonia. In this stage, the involved lobe is often covered with fibrin. The cut surface is gray, dry, and granular. The alveoli are uniformly filled throughout the lobe with a fibrinous network and neutrophils. Alveolar walls are remarkably intact. Complications of lobar pneumonia include pleural effusion; fibrinous pleuritis; empyema and fibrinous or fibrinopurulent pericarditis; and acute otitis media.

Bronchopneumonia is usually secondary to chronic passive congestion of the lungs, aspiration, debilitation, or some disease of the respiratory tract such as influenza. Plugging of the bronchi with mucus is an important factor in the pathogenesis. The most common causes of bronchopneumonia are coagulase-positive <u>Staphylococcus</u> <u>aureus</u> and gram-negative bacteria such as <u>Pseudomonas</u> <u>aeruginosa</u>, Klebsiella-Aerobacter group, and <u>Escherichia</u> <u>coli</u>.

On palpation of the lungs in bronchopneumonia, foci of increased resistance are felt. These vary from grayish yellow to dark red. The foci are patchy and mainly located around small bronchi and bronchioles. Abscess formation is common in cases of bronchopneumonia. The bronchial lumina are filled with neutrophils. Their walls are edematous, congested, and infiltrated by neutrophils. The alveoli surrounding the bronchi and bronchioles are filled with neutrophils, eosinophilic fluid, fibrin, and macrophages.

Acute interstitial pneumonia may be produced by <u>Coxiella</u> <u>burnetii</u> and influenza viruses. Most of the cases in which cold agglutinins are found are caused by <u>Mycoplasma</u> <u>pneumoniae</u>. The lungs typically show patchy foci of consolidation. The alveolar septa are infiltrated by lymphocytes and macrophages, and are edematous. Hyaline membranes line the alveolar walls.

Legionellosis is caused by <u>Legionella</u> <u>pneumophila</u>. It usually occurs in outbreaks among older persons, especially men and cigarette smokers. Spread is airborne from contaminated air conditioning water systems, streams, or newly dug soil. Person to person spread is unusual. Alveoli and respiratory bronchioles are filled with neutrophils, macrophages, and fibrin. Legionellosis often develops in immunosuppressed patients.

Bronchiectasis signifies a permanent dilatation of the bronchi, usually associated with suppuration. The lower lobes are involved more often than the upper. In most instances, several causes act together to produce the bronchial dilatation. Some form of bronchial obstruction is often noted proximal to the dilatation. Infection is usually combined with obstruction, each accentuating the other. Bronchial infection without obstruction may cause bronchiectasis in some cases, as in pertussis. In mucoviscidosis, bronchiectasis is a common feature, due to bronchial obstruction from viscid mucus production.

In bronchiectasis the bronchi are dilated, thin-walled, and often distended with pus. The bronchial walls show a relative reduction in muscular and elastic elements. Ciliated bronchial epithelium is often replaced by squamous epithelium promoting stagnation. Increased vascularity of the affected lobes is almost always noted, due to the development of shunts between the bronchial and pulmonary arteries. Pulmonary hypertension leads to the development of chronic cor pulmonale.

Lung abscess is a localized area of tissue destruction and suppuration within the lung parenchyma. Mixed bacterial infections are common, with anaerobic and saprophytic organisms predominating; occasionally fungi are responsible. Aspiration of a foreign body often precedes the development of lung abscess. Septic embolism usually produces multiple bilateral septic infarcts or abscesses. Lung abscess may also follow bland pulmonary embolism; the ischemic or infarcted lung tissue breaks down and forms an abscess when secondarily infected from the bronchial tree. Lung abscess may follow staphylococcal or gram-negative pneumonia. Bronchogenic carcinoma should be suspected in adults when signs of abscess develop without apparent cause.

In acute abscess, as following aspiration of vomitus and rapid bacterial invasion, a large segment of lung may be hemorrhagic and indurated and show a ragged cavity filled with sanguinopurulent material. Most lung abscesses are chronic. The affected lung shows a shrunken lobe covered with dense adhesions. On section there is a airless, fibrotic zone surrounding a cavity containing pus and communicating with a bronchus. This cavity is lined with granulation tissue and heavily infiltrated with leukocytes. Usually the abscess ruptures into a bronchus, if there was no such communication at the beginning. Rupture into the pleural sac is also common, producing empyema, pneumothorax, and bronchopleural fistula. Brain abscess may complicate any of the chronic suppurative lesions such as lung abscess, bronchiectasis, and empyema. Secondary amyloidosis may also complicate chronic pulmonary suppuration.

278. A 50 year-old man who had smoked over a pack of cigarettes daily for many years had a hacking cough productive of mucoid sputum for 2 years. He had scattered rhonchi and wheezing. The likeliest diagnosis is

   (A)   asthma
   (B)   bronchiectasis
   (C)   chronic bronchitis
   (D)   chronic pneumonitis
   (E)   diffuse pulmonary fibrosis

279. All of the following are characteristic of the disease diagnosed in Item 278 **EXCEPT**:

   (A)   bacteria play an important role in its causation
   (B)   bronchial walls are infiltrated by lymphocytes and macrophages
   (C)   bronchial walls show smooth muscle hypertrophy
   (D)   bronchial mucous glands are hyperplastic
   (E)   the Reid index is increased

280. All of the following are characteristic of asthma **EXCEPT**:

   (A)   bronchial mucous glands are hyperplastic
   (B)   bronchial walls are infiltrated by eosinophils
   (C)   bronchial walls show smooth muscle hypertrophy
   (D)   foci of squamous metaplasia develop on bronchial mucosa
   (E)   the Reid index is increased

In Items 281-286, match each item with the type or types of emphysema to which it is most closely related.

   (A)   centrilobular emphysema
   (B)   panlobular emphysema
   (C)   both
   (D)   neither

281. α_1-antitrypsin deficiency

282. chronic bronchitis

283. cigarette smoking

284. involvement of pulmonary acini

285.   occurs most often in older men

286.   pulmonary scar

ANSWERS AND TUTORIAL ON ITEMS 278-286

The answers are: **278-C; 279-A; 280-D; 281-B; 282-A; 283-C; 284-C; 285-A; 286-D**.

Chronic bronchitis is one of the most common respiratory diseases due to cigarette smoking. While bacteria are sometimes present in foci of chronic bronchitis they are not a primary causative factor. Chronic bronchitis is one of the chronic obstructive lung diseases, the others being asthma, emphysema, and diffuse bronchiectasis.

In Item 278, the smoking history and productive hacking cough for at least 2 years is indicative of chronic bronchitis.

Despite their totally different causation, the bronchi in asthma and chronic bronchitis share many similarities microscopically. Both show large amounts of mucus, mucous gland hyperplasia, smooth muscle hypertrophy, and thickening of the basement membrane. Eosinophils are present in asthma, and squamous metaplasia in chronic bronchitis.

In Items 281-286, an α_1-antitrypsin deficiency predisposes to some cases of panlobular emphysema; chronic bronchitis and occurrence in older men are more closely related to centrilobular emphysema; cigarette smoking and involvement of respiratory acini are associated with both forms. Pulmonary scars are associated with irregular emphysema.

In chronic bronchitis mucus is often found in the lumen of the bronchi, and the bronchial mucosal glands are hyperplastic. The bronchial walls are somewhat thickened by fibrosis and smooth muscular hypertrophy. In the submucosa, there is an infiltration of lymphocytes and macrophages. There may be foci of squamous metaplasia of the bronchial epithelium, and the epithelial basement membrane is thickened. The Reid index (the ratio of the width of bronchial mucous glands to the thickness of the bronchial wall, normally less than 0.36), is increased to 0.41 - 0.79.

In asthma the larger bronchi contain large amounts of mucus, and the mucosa is edematous and injected. The walls of medium-sized and small bronchi are thickened, and their lumina are narrowed and filled with tenacious mucus. Goblet cell metaplasia of the surface mucosal cells occurs. There are thickening and hyalinization of the epithelial basement membrane in the medium-sized bronchi. The submucosa shows moderate fibrosis and eosinophilic infiltration. Bronchial mucous glands are hyperplastic and are often distended with mucus. The Reid index is increased.

Emphysema is an irreversible over-distention and destruction of pulmonary acini. In centrilobular emphysema, the respiratory bronchioles are dilated and destroyed. The upper lobes are mainly involved. There is a strong association with chronic bronchitis and cigarette smoking. Older men are most often affected. In panlobular (panacinar) emphysema, the entire acinus is involved and the entire lung is diffusely affected. Men and women are about equally affected, and there is a causal association with cigarette smoking. Some cases are due to a deficiency of

α_1-antitrypsin, especially in women. Grossly in emphysema the lungs are voluminous and feathery. An emphysematous bulla may rupture, causing pneumothorax.

Items 287-291

287. Progressive massive fibrosis of the lungs occurs in

   (A)   coal worker's pneumoconiosis
   (B)   healed tuberculosis
   (C)   organized pneumonia
   (D)   radiation pneumonitis
   (E)   sarcoidosis

288. Of the following, the lung disorder which is most characteristically associated with the development of pulmonary tuberculosis is

   (A)   anthracosis
   (B)   bronchiectasis
   (C)   centrilobular emphysema
   (D)   lipid pneumonia
   (E)   silicosis

289. Immunologic diseases of the lungs include all of the following **EXCEPT**:

   (A)   chronic berylliosis
   (B)   extrinsic asthma
   (C)   farmer's lung
   (D)   Goodpasture's syndrome
   (E)   silicosis

290. The cause of farmer's lung is

   (A)   hypersensitivity to actinomycetes in moldy hay
   (B)   hypersensitivity to actinomycetes in bagasse
   (C)   hypersensitivity to antigen in bird droppings
   (D)   hypersensitivity to antigen in wheat weevil
   (E)   nitrogen dioxide in silage

110

291. Diffuse interstitial pulmonary fibrosis may be caused by all of the following **EXCEPT**:

(A) busulfan therapy
(B) chronic extrinsic hypersensitivity alveolitis
(C) organization of lobar pneumonia
(D) pneumoconiosis
(E) usual interstitial pneumonitis

ANSWERS AND TUTORIAL ON ITEMS 287-291

The answers are: **287-A; 288-E; 289-E; 290-A; 291-C**.

Coal worker's pneumoconiosis (CWP, black lung disease), is characterized by the formation of interstitial nodules of anthracotic pigment with associated fibrosis. It may lead to massive fibrosis of the lungs. Silicosis is associated with an increased incidence of tuberculosis (miner's phthisis) as well as of bronchogenic carcinoma.

The lungs are the site of a host of immunologic diseases due to inhaled or circulating allergens. The offending agent in farmer's lung is a thermophilic actinomycete, Micropolyspora faeni. This is also the cause of extrinsic hypersensitivity alveolitis. Actinomycetes (M. vulgaris) also cause bagassosis, due to inhalation of sugar cane residue dust. Nitrogen dioxide from nitrates in corn causes silo-filler's lung.

In Item 291, organized pneumonia is focal. Usual interstitial pneumonitis is an idiopathic pulmonary fibrosis.

Pneumoconiosis is a collective term for the pathologic changes caused by particulate matter inhaled into the lungs. Most cases of pneumoconiosis are occupational in origin, occurring among miners and processers of certain harmful substances. Anthracosis is the deposition in the lungs of black coal pigment.

Silicosis is caused by the deposition of silica particles which have been inhaled into the lungs. When silica particles 0.5 - 5 μm in diameter enter an alveolus, they are immediately phagocytized by macrophages which die and attract neutrophils and more macrophages. The latter become epithelioid cells, and later giant cells are formed. Fibroblastic proliferation leads to formation of the silicotic nodule. Collagen is laid down, and the epithelioid cells and most giant cells disappear. Throughout the lungs numerous firm, spherical, grayish white nodules 1 to 3 mm. in diameter are found. The nodules consist of whorls of hyalinized fibrous tissue containing pigment granules. The silicotic nodules are discrete early, but they eventually coalesce, producing widespread fibrosis. Emphysema is common about the nodules.

Asbestosis occurs among the workers who handle asbestos-containing materials. The asbestos body is produced by the deposition of protein and iron pigment from the inflammatory exudate upon the surface of the asbestos fiber. The lungs are firm and nodular. There is a diffuse fibrosis, especially about bronchioles. Within the fibrous tissue are the characteristic asbestos bodies, which are golden yellow, segmented, and globular. The incidence of bronchogenic carcinoma and mesothelioma is increased in asbestos-exposed workers.

In idiopathic diffuse interstitial pulmonary fibrosis (usual interstitial pneumonitis, UIP), diffuse fibrosis develops within a month of the onset of symptoms and may cause death within six months. However, some cases become chronic. The disease is uncommon and occurs most often in middle-aged adults. Dyspnea and cyanosis are prominent. Several cases have followed influenzal pneumonia.

Items 292-297

292. Local complications due to bronchial obstruction by a bronchogenic carcinoma include all of the following **EXCEPT**:

(A) atelectasis
(B) bronchiectasis
(C) bronchopneumonia
(D) emphysema
(E) lung abscess

293. Metabolic abnormalities associated with bronchogenic adenoma or carcinoma include all of the following **EXCEPT**:

(A) carcinoid syndrome
(B) Cushing's syndrome
(C) hypercalcemia
(D) hypoglycemia
(E) inappropriate antidiuretic hormone secretion

294. A 50 year-old woman had had tuberculosis involving the left upper lobe years ago. It had been treated successfully with isoniazid, but there was considerable residual fibrosis. A carcinoma had developed in the LUL. The type of lung cancer most often associated with pulmonary scars is

(A) adenocarcinoma
(B) anaplastic small cell carcinoma
(C) epidermoid carcinoma
(D) giant cell carcinoma
(E) metastatic carcinoma

A 60 year-old man, who had been a heavy smoker for years, noted weight loss, dyspnea, and coughing. Bronchoscopy revealed a mass in the right main bronchus. A photomicrograph of the biopsy is shown in Figure 4.2.

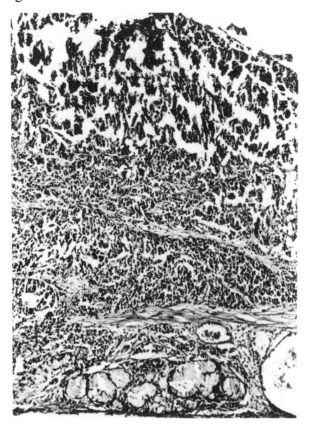

Figure 4.2

295.   The likeliest diagnosis is

    (A)   anaplastic small cell carcinoma
    (B)   carcinoid bronchial adenoma
    (C)   lymphoma
    (D)   poorly differentiated adenocarcinoma
    (E)   squamous cell carcinoma

296. Common sites of metastases from primary lung cancer include all of the following **EXCEPT**:

   (A)   adrenal glands
   (B)   bones
   (C)   brain
   (D)   liver
   (E)   spleen

297. A 60 year-old man developed pain down the right arm and ipsilateral Horner's syndrome. The likeliest cause is

   (A)   apical lung abscess
   (B)   metastatic carcinoma in lower cervical lymph nodes
   (C)   pulmonary scar carcinoma in apex
   (D)   reinfection apical tuberculosis
   (E)   superior pulmonary sulcus carcinoma (Pancoast tumor)

ANSWERS AND TUTORIAL ON ITEMS 292-297

The answers are: **292-D; 293-D; 294-A; 295-A; 296-E; 297-E.**

Sometimes lung cancers are diagnosed because of complications they cause by bronchial obstruction. These may produce signs of an infection or be noted on a routine chest film.

Bronchogenic carcinomas, especially anaplastic small cell ones, may cause a paraneoplastic syndrome by secreting a hormone. Bronchial adenoma of the carcinoid type, which is really a low grade malignant tumor, produces serotonin. Small cell carcinomas secrete ACTH and antidiuretic hormone, and epidermoid carcinoma releases parathormone.

In Item 294, scar carcinoma is usually an adenocarcinoma, and in Item 297, the superior pulmonary sulcus tumor is usually a squamous one. It invades the brachial plexus and lower cervical sympathetic ganglia.

Most bronchogenic carcinomas have metastasized by the time they are discovered, either via lymphatics or hematogenously. The adrenals are a common metastatic site, as are the brain, liver, bones, and kidneys.

Epidermoid carcinoma, the most common type of bronchogenic carcinoma, arises from metaplastic squamous epithelium of main stem bronchi or the next subdivision, and constitutes about 40 percent of all bronchogenic carcinomas. Spread is chiefly by extension to hilar lymph nodes, chest wall, and mediastinum. Cigarette smoking is the most important causative factor, as it is with anaplastic small cell and many adenocarcinomas of bronchi.

Anaplastic small cell (oat cell) carcinoma may arise from pulmonary endocrine cells, especially of the main stem bronchi, and comprises about 20 percent of all bronchogenic carcinomas. It is more common in men than in women. Microscopically this neoplasm is

114

composed of small cells resembling lymphocytes, with scanty cytoplasm and darkly staining nuclei. Distant hematogenous spread is common.

Adenocarcinoma arises from the epithelial cells of the bronchial surface or glands. This tumor comprises about 30 percent of all lung carcinomas and affects both sexes about equally. It is generally located more peripherally in the bronchial tree than the other types. Microscopically it is composed of gland-forming mucin-secreting epithelial cells. Its spread is chiefly by the blood stream. Bronchiolo-alveolar carcinoma (pulmonary adenomatosis) arises in the epithelium of terminal bronchioles and grows slowly, rarely producing bronchial obstruction. Grossly this neoplasm resembles in some cases the uniform consolidation of lobar pneumonia; in other cases it is multicentric in origin. Microscopically groups of alveoli are lined with tall, clear mucin-secreting cells. Metastasis is largely confined to the hilar nodes.

Pulmonary scar carcinoma arises in fibrous scar resulting from chronic pneumonitis, an abscess, bronchiectasis, or tuberculosis. Most of these neoplasms are peripheral, and the overlying pleura is puckered. Such carcinomas arise from bronchiolar epithelium, and histologically most are adenocarcinoma.

The special manifestations of the superior pulmonary sulcus tumor (Pancoast tumor) are dependent upon location at or adjoining the thoracic inlet. Infiltration of the brachial plexus gives pain and muscle atrophy in an arm; involvement of the cervical sympathetic chain causes Horner's syndrome; and compression of the superior vena cava results in edema of the face and upper extremities (superior vena cava syndrome).

Metastatic neoplasms of the lungs and pleura are more common than primary neoplasms. Such metastases occur in about 25 percent of all fatal malignant neoplasms. The most common neoplasms giving rise to pulmonary or pleural metastases are carcinoma of the breast, gastrointestinal tract, kidneys, and malignant melanoma. Neoplastic cells may reach the lung by direct extension, pulmonary arterial embolism, or retrograde lymphatic extension from the mediastinal lymph nodes. Metastatic neoplasms in the lungs are typically multiple and bilateral. When they are in the parenchyma of the lungs, they are usually rounded. When spread is by lymphatic channels, the pleura often shows thread-like extensions of tumor.

Items 298-300

298.   Adult respiratory distress syndrome (ARDS) occurs in all of the following **EXCEPT**:

      (A)   brain injuries
      (B)   heroin overdose
      (C)   high oxygen concentrations on respirator
      (D)   pulmonary embolism
      (E)   shock

299.   Atelectasis may be due to all of the following **EXCEPT**:

(A)   bronchiectasis
(B)   inhaled foreign body in bronchus
(C)   mucus plugs in bronchi
(D)   pleural effusion
(E)   spontaneous pneumothorax

300.   The causes of pulmonary hypertension include all of the following **EXCEPT**:

(A)   diffuse pulmonary fibrosis
(B)   emphysema of lungs
(C)   multiple small pulmonary emboli
(D)   mitral stenosis
(E)   tetralogy of Fallot

ANSWERS AND TUTORIAL ON ITEMS 298-300

The answers are: **298-D; 299-A; 300-E**. Adult respiratory distress syndrome (ARDS) is characterized by severe pulmonary edema unrelated to left ventricular failure, with resulting acute respiratory failure. Among its many causes are shock, including that due to burns, gram-negative sepsis, and acute pancreatitis; exposure to toxic gases, including high oxygen concentrations; heroin or barbiturate overdoses; uremia; drowning; disseminated intravascular coagulation; and brain injuries. The underlying mechanism is damage to the alveolar walls with resultant increased permeability. The alveoli are filled with edema fluid and lined by fibrinous hyaline membranes. Later, if the patient survives, there is a proliferative phase, sometimes with intra-alveolar and interstitial fibrosis.

Atelectasis is a collapsed state of all or a part of a lung. At birth both lungs are atelectatic (primary atelectasis). With the onset of respiration, the alveoli expand. Secondary atelectasis includes any collapse of the alveoli after the primary expansion in neonatal life has taken place.

Compression atelectasis is due to extrinsic pressure on all or part of a lung driving the air out and producing collapse. It is complete when the pressure is great and uniform, as in a large pleural effusion, empyema, or pneumothorax. Obstructive atelectasis is due to complete blockage of a bronchus caused by a neoplastic mass, mucus, or an inhaled foreign body. The air distal to the block is absorbed, leading to collapse of the involved portion of the lung.

Primary pulmonary hypertension occurs most commonly in women between the ages of 20 and 40. Significant changes are found in the small muscular arteries and arterioles which show concentric intimal fibroblastic proliferation and deposition of mucopolysaccharide with luminal narrowing or obliteration. In the media, smooth muscle hypertrophy may be found.

Secondary pulmonary hypertension is usually due to increased pulmonary arterial pressure and/or flow. Some cases are due to the organization of multiple emboli or thrombi in small pulmonary arteries and arterioles. Secondary pulmonary hypertension occurs in cases of congenital heart disease with left-to-right shunt; mitral stenosis; diffuse pulmonary fibrosis; emphysema; multiple pulmonary emboli; kyphoscoliosis; and systemic hypertension. Chronic cor pulmonale develops in most cases of secondary pulmonary sclerosis and hypertension. The right ventricular myocardium is hypertrophied, and the ventricle is frequently dilated. A secondary polycythemia commonly develops.

CHAPTER V

DIGESTIVE SYSTEM PATHOLOGY

Items 301-305

301. A 60 year-old man developed gradually increasing difficulty in swallowing, first to solid foods, then to liquids. Endoscopic examination and barium swallow revealed an esophageal carcinoma at the lower end. All of the following are true statements concerning esophageal cancer **EXCEPT**:

 (A)   alcohol and cigarette smoking are causative factors
 (B)   a fistula may develop from the esophagus to a bronchus
 (C)   adenocarcinoma may develop at the lower end of the esophagus
 (D)   carcinoma of the upper end may occur in the Plummer-Vinson syndrome
 (E)   death is usually due to metastases to lungs and liver

302. A 30 year-old salesman developed sharp epigastric pain relieved by eating. An upper G-I series demonstrated a 1 cm. duodenal ulcer. The most important factor in the development of peptic ulcer of the duodenum is

 (A)   decreased mucosal resistance
 (B)   gastrin secreting islet cell adenoma
 (C)   having group O blood
 (D)   hypersecretion of gastric hydrochloric acid
 (E)   prolonged adrenocorticosteroid therapy

303. Peptic ulcer may occur in all of the following **EXCEPT**:

 (A)   lower esophagus
 (B)   stomach
 (C)   jejunum
 (D)   ileum adjacent to Meckel's diverticulum
 (E)   cecum

304. Major complications of duodenal peptic ulcer include all of the following **EXCEPT**:

(A) hemorrhage
(B) malignant transformation
(C) obstruction
(D) perforation

305. Factors associated with an increased incidence of carcinoma of the stomach include all of the following **EXCEPT**:

(A) eating fish or other foods salted with nitrates
(B) gastric polyps
(C) group A blood
(D) hypertrophic pyloric stenosis
(E) pernicious anemia

ANSWERS AND TUTORIAL ON ITEMS 301-305

The answers are: **301-E; 302-D; 303-E; 304-B; 305-D**. Carcinoma of the esophagus is more common in males than in females. Alcoholism and smoking are contributory etiologic factors. Most patients with esophageal cancer are over age 50. Carcinomas of the esophagus begin as flat nodules in the mucosa and spread in the submucosa, slowly encircling the esophagus and narrowing the lumen. A fistula through the tumor area may form between a bronchus and the esophagus. Direct extension to the mediastinum and lung may occur. About 90 percent are epidermoid carcinoma. Occasionally adenocarcinoma arises in the lower end from ectopic gastric glands. Distant metastasis is unusual in carcinoma of the esophagus.

The Plummer-Vinson syndrome, consisting of dysphagia plus hypochromic microcytic anemia, is a disorder of middle-aged women. An esophageal ring (web) may form in the upper esophagus. The syndrome is sometimes complicated years later by epidermoid carcinoma of the upper end of the esophagus.

Peptic ulcer is chronic and may occur in the lower esophagus, stomach, duodenum, jejunum, or adjacent to a Meckel's diverticulum. Almost all develop along the lesser curvature in the antral portion of the stomach or within the first 2 cm. of the duodenum. It is more common in men than women by about 3:1, and duodenal ulcer is especially frequent in men. Duodenal ulcer is especially common in persons with group O blood. The major complications of duodenal peptic ulcer are perforation (the main cause of death), hemorrhage, and obstruction at or near the pylorus. Development of malignant change in a benign ulcer is rare.

An important cause of peptic ulcer is the hypersecretion of gastric hydrochloric acid, especially with duodenal ulcers. Gastric ulcer may occur in patients with normal or even decreased gastric acid, probably due to decreased mucosal resistance. Recurring and intractable peptic ulceration, usually of the duodenum but also of the jejunum and stomach, may be associated with islet cell tumors of the pancreas (Zollinger-Ellison syndrome). Gastrin secretion by these tumors leads to increased gastric acid production. Patients under long-term steroid therapy are prone to develop peptic ulcer. Those using aspirin or nonsteroidal anti-inflammatory agents have an increased incidence of ulcers.

About 85 percent of all peptic ulcers occur in the duodenum, chiefly in the first part (the duodenal bulb). Most of the rest occur in the stomach, usually within 5 cm. of the pylorus and on or near the lesser curvature. Peptic ulcers are single in about 90 percent of the cases. Most are 1 to 2.5 cm. in diameter. The edges are usually sharply punched out, and the base consists of muscularis with a thin covering of scar tissue and exudate.

Benign neoplasms of the stomach are uncommon and include leiomyoma and adenoma. Adenomas, usually in the form of multiple adenomatous polyps (gastric polyposis), are important because they can become malignant.

Carcinoma of the stomach is more common in men than women. Most cases occur after age 40. Gastric carcinoma is several times more frequent in patients with pernicious anemia than in the general population. It occurs more commonly in persons with group A blood than the expected rate.

Carcinoma of the stomach occurs in high incidence in Japan, Chile, and Iceland apparently due to increased ingestion of nitrates which are converted to nitrites and nitrosamines. Pickled and salted fish or beans and high nitrate content in soil and water are sources of dietary nitrate.

Three general forms of stomach cancer are recognized grossly: a fungating growth which bulges into the lumen of the stomach and which may arise from an adenomatous polyp; ulcerating carcinoma which has raised, indurated edges and an ulcer crater for a base; and infiltrating carcinoma, which causes a marked thickening of the wall of the stomach. Most gastric carcinoma is adenocarcinoma.

Items 306-310

306.   The major cause of sprue in the U.S. is

     (A)   bacterial infection
     (B)   deficiency of vitamin B_{12}
     (C)   hypersensitivity to gliadin fraction of wheat gluten
     (D)   lymphatic obstruction
     (E)   pancreatic insufficiency

307. A 20 year-old man complained of intermittent diarrhea and lower abdominal pain. An upper G-I series showed segmental narrowing in the ileum. The likeliest diagnosis is

   (A)   adenocarcinoma
   (B)   carcinoid
   (C)   intestinal lipodystrophy (Whipple's disease)
   (D)   regional enteritis (Crohn's disease)
   (E)   tuberculosis

308. All of the following are characteristic of the disease in Item 307 **EXCEPT**:

   (A)   association with arthritis and uveitis
   (B)   fistula formation between loops of intestine
   (C)   frequent perforation of involved intestine with peritonitis
   (D)   granulomatous reaction in all layers of involved intestine
   (E)   skip areas between involved segments of intestine

309. All of the following are characteristic of Whipple's disease **EXCEPT**:

   (A)   it is caused by an unidentified bacterium
   (B)   it is a malabsorption syndrome for lipids
   (C)   mesenteric lymph nodes show a granulomatous reaction
   (D)   there is an increased incidence of small intestinal adenocarcinoma
   (E)   vacuolated macrophages containing lipid and glycoprotein are found in the jejunum and ileum

310. A 30 year-old woman had episodes of flushing of the face, nausea, and diarrhea. At surgery a yellow tumor was found in the wall of the ileum. The most likely diagnosis of the tumor is

   (A)   adenoma
   (B)   adenocarcinoma
   (C)   carcinoid
   (D)   leiomyoma
   (E)   mucoepidermoid carcinoma

ANSWERS AND TUTORIAL ON ITEMS 306-310

The answers are: **306-C; 307-D; 308-C; 309-D; 310-C.** Sprue (gluten-induced enteropathy, celiac disease) is a complex deficiency state which occurs in infants or young or middle-aged adults and presents as a syndrome of malnutrition resulting from defective intestinal absorption. There is usually megaloblastic anemia due to insufficient absorption of vitamin B_{12}. Gluten-induced enteropathy is due to a defect in small intestinal enzymatic activity accentuated by the ingestion of wheat gluten. Patients have high titers of anti-gliadin antibodies and increased serum levels of IgA. Gluten-induced sprue has an increased frequency in persons with histocompatibility antigen HLA 8. It may be inherited as a dominant with incomplete penetrance.

Regional enteritis (Crohn's disease) is an idiopathic chronic inflammatory disease, common in young adults, characterized by hose-like thickening of the distal portion of the small intestine. An abnormal immunologic reaction is suspected because of the fairly frequent association of arthritis, uveitis, and erythema nodosum of the skin with regional enteritis. The terminal ileum is usually affected, but the jejunum and duodenum are sometimes involved. The colon is involved in about 25 percent of cases, especially perianally. Usually only one segment of the bowel suffers, but involvement of separate segments may be noted. The affected segments of intestine are sharply demarcated from healthy bowel, thickened, gray-red, and stiff as a garden hose. The lumen of the bowel becomes greatly reduced in size as the walls become thickened by edema. In acute cases, an exudate consisting largely of macrophages and eosinophils appears in the tissue spaces. In chronic cases, there is a granulomatous reaction in all layers of the bowel and mesentery, affecting especially the lacteals. The lesions in the submucosa, mesentery, and lymph nodes may resemble sarcoidosis very closely. Fistulas are common. There is an increase in small intestinal adenocarcinoma, especially in the ileum, in patients with Crohn's disease.

Intestinal lipodystrophy (Whipple's disease) is caused by an unidentified bacterium. Whipple's disease is a malabsorption syndrome, there being almost complete failure to absorb lipids. The disease usually occurs in males at about age 50. Grossly the mucosal folds of the jejunum and ileum show yellowish foci and dilated lacteals. Numerous vacuolated macrophages containing glycoprotein are present in the lamina propria. Lipid is demonstrated intercellularly and within macrophages in the lamina propria. Electron-dense, sickle-shaped particles within macrophages and extracellularly are probably bacteria. The mesenteric lymph nodes may be yellow and contain much fat which incites a granulomatous reaction with macrophages and occasionally foreign-body giant cells.

Primary neoplasms of the small intestine are rare. Carcinoid tumors, although uncommon, are the most frequent primary neoplasms of the small intestine. They may be evident grossly as one or more yellow, submucosal nodules, growing slowly and infiltrating locally. Carcinoids arise from neural crest (Kulchitsky) cells and may occur in bronchi, gastrointestinal tract, or pancreas. Microscopically, the carcinoid shows nests of polyhedral cells, resembling closely the islet cells of the pancreas, embedded in a fibrous stroma. In about 20 percent of the cases, carcinoids of the small intestine metastasize, usually to the liver. When there are large masses of functioning carcinoid there is an increase in serotonin in the blood, resulting in episodic crises of skin flushing, nausea, and diarrhea (carcinoid syndrome). Peculiar fibrous tissue deposits (fibrostenosis) may occur in the pulmonary and tricuspid valves, leading to cor pulmonale.

311. A 25 year-old woman developed diarrhea, abdominal pain, and rectal bleeding. Sigmoidoscopy showed numerous ulcers, and the diagnosis of ulcerative colitis was made. All of the following are characteristic of ulcerative colitis **EXCEPT**:

    (A) association with arthritis, uveitis, and biliary cirrhosis
    (B) crypt abscess formation deep in mucosa
    (C) frequent perforation of ulcers with peritonitis
    (D) increased incidence of adenocarcinoma of colon
    (E) pseudopolyp formation between ulcers

312. The commonest complication of diverticulosis of the colon is

    (A) development of carcinoma
    (B) diverticulitis
    (C) hemorrhage
    (D) obstruction
    (E) perforation

313. Of the following acute peritonitis is **LEAST** likely to occur in a case of

    (A) acute appendicitis
    (B) acute cholecystitis
    (C) colonic diverticulitis
    (D) duodenal ulcer
    (E) intestinal lipodystrophy

314. Factors associated with an increased incidence of carcinoma of the colon include all of the following **EXCEPT**:

    (A) familial colonic polyposis
    (B) cholecystectomy
    (C) low fiber, high fat diet
    (D) Peutz-Jeghers syndrome
    (E) ulcerative colitis

315. Causes of intestinal obstruction include all of the following **EXCEPT**:

    (A)   acute peritonitis
    (B)   carcinoma of sigmoid colon
    (C)   intussusception
    (D)   carcinoma of cecum
    (E)   volvulus

A 60 year-old man developed obstinate constipation. A barium enema revealed an obstructive lesion in the sigmoid colon. Surgery was performed. A photograph of the gross specimen in shown in Figure 5.1.

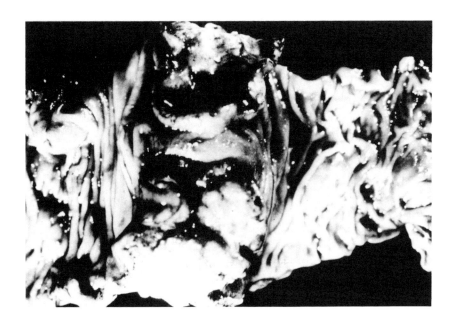

Figure 5.1

316. The likeliest diagnosis is

    (A)   adenocarcinoma
    (B)   adenomatous polyp
    (C)   carcinoid
    (D)   diverticulitis
    (E)   pseudomembranous colitis

ANSWERS AND TUTORIAL ON ITEMS 311-316

The answers are: 311-C; 312-B; 313-E; 314-D; 315-D; 316-A. Ulcerative colitis is an idiopathic inflammatory disease of the colon characterized by ulceration and scarring. Most cases have their onset between the ages of 20 and 40 years. Antibodies against mucopolysaccharide in colonic mucosal cells are found in most patients. A delayed hypersensitivity reaction also appears to be involved. The sigmoid colon is most commonly affected. In the earliest stages, the mucosa shows scattered hemorrhages and marked hyperemia. Later the mucosa is irregularly ulcerated, leaving strips and islands of intact mucosa. If ulceration is shallow, there is a cobblestone effect; if deep, the patches of mucosa between the ulcers stand out prominently (pseudopolyps). Crypt abscesses are noted deep in the mucosa. These dissect in the submucosa and rupture onto the surface. Arthritis, uveitis, erythema nodosum, and biliary cirrhosis are commonly associated. Perforation with peritonitis is rare, but is the most common cause of death in fatal cases. Colonic carcinoma develops in about 5 percent of cases of long duration.

A diverticulum of the intestine is a mural outpouching whose mucosal lining is continuous with that of the intestine. If multiple diverticula are present, as is common in the acquired form, the condition is diverticulosis. If one or more diverticula become inflamed, the process is diverticulitis. Acquired diverticula are usually multiple. They are most common in elderly persons, especially those subject to constipation. A low residue diet which leads to excessive segmental colonic contraction has been implicated as the cause. Diverticula are most common in the sigmoid colon where they bulge between the longitudinal muscle bands.

When a fecalith forms in a diverticulum, drainage from the pocket may be blocked, and pathogenic bacteria may penetrate the mucosa, giving rise to diverticulitis, the most common complication of diverticulosis. In acute cases, perforation may occur, causing peritonitis, but usually diverticulitis is more chronic, causing much peridiverticular inflammation and fibrosis. This may lead to chronic intestinal obstruction.

Acute diffuse peritonitis is usually of either chemical or bacterial origin. Chemical peritonitis may be a result of acute pancreatitis or of perforation of the gallbladder or stomach. Bacterial peritonitis is much more common. It usually results from rupture of or extension from, a diseased hollow viscus within the peritoneal cavity: appendix; gallbladder; intestinal diverticulum; perforated ulcer, as with typhoid fever, ulcerative colitis, and peptic ulcer; intestinal obstruction; gonorrheal salpingitis; puerperal endometritis; or penetrating injury.

In acute peritonitis, the peritoneal cavity contains a serous, fibrinous, purulent, or sanguineous exudate, depending upon the nature and duration of the infection. Fibrin is almost constantly present giving a granular appearance to the serosal surface and binding adjacent loops of intestine to each other. The intestine becomes distended due to paralytic ileus.

Adenomatous polyps and villous adenomas of the colon are more numerous in men than women and are often multiple. Most colonic polyps are found in the recto-sigmoid portion. They are usually 0.1 to 5.0 cm. in diameter. They may have a broad base or a long pedicle. They show piling up of the epithelium, cell atypism, loss of cell polarity, and frequent mitotic figures. In familial multiple polyposis, many adenomatous polyps averaging 1 cm. in diameter develop in the colon between the ages of 10 and 30. There is a high incidence of malignant transformation of one or more of the polyps by 40 years of age. The Peutz-Jeghers syndrome

126

consists of melanin pigmentation of the lips and buccal mucosa with multiple hamartomatous gastrointestinal polyps, especially in the small intestine. These polyps rarely undergo malignant change.

Carcinoma of the colon (including the rectum) is one of the most common forms of malignant neoplasm in both men and women. Nearly three-fourths of all cancers of the colon occur in the rectosigmoid portion. Circulating carcinoembryonic antigen (CEA) can be detected in patients with colonic carcinoma. Early lesions often show a polypoid, intraluminal growth. The tumor can extend around the bowel in an annular fashion, narrowing the lumen. Ulceration is common and may be deep. In early cases, the tumor is limited to the wall of the bowel (Group A of Duke's staging); later it extends into the serosal tissues (group B); finally regional lymph node and distant metastases occur (group C). Microscopically the neoplasm is composed of glandular epithelium (adenocarcinoma).

The cause of colon and rectal carcinoma is unknown. It is a disease of the Western industrialized countries. Low-fiber diet has been causally implicated. Increased dietary fat has also been blamed, especially in relation to the possible conversion of bile acids and cholesterol to carcinogens by anaerobic bacteria in the colon. Some cases of colon cancer occur in cases of ulcerative colitis and inherited colonic polyposis. A few cases have developed in women who have received radiation therapy for uterine cancer. Persons who have had cholecystectomies are at increased risk of developing colon cancer, especially in the right colon. This may be related to changes in concentrations of bile acids in the bile of patients without a gallbladder.

Intestinal obstruction may be a result of kinking of the tube, blockage of the lumen, or failure of the driving force. The first two are commonly spoken of as organic obstruction, the third as paralytic.

Kinking of the intestine usually causes sudden and complete intestinal obstruction. It is most commonly due to trapping of a mobile loop, usually jejunum or ileum since their mesentery is longest, in a narrow, preformed pocket known as a hernial sac. Sometimes violent peristalsis will cause a twisting of the intestine on its mesentery, often at the site of a peritoneal adhesion. This volvulus occurs most frequently in elderly persons; it causes venous obstruction and gangrene of the strangulated segment of bowel if it is not corrected.

The lumen of the intestine may be blocked as a result of tissue changes in the wall of the intestine, or by abnormal structures in the lumen. Obstruction of this sort is usually gradual in onset, and only slowly becomes complete. Neoplasms of the intestine comprise the most important segment of this group. However, cecal carcinoma rarely causes obstruction because it grows as a polypoid mass in a large tube in which the contents are liquid. Chronic inflammatory diseases of the intestine, such as regional enteritis and lymphopathia venereum, may cause strictures of the intestine. Rarely do foreign bodies cause blockage of the lumen. When they do, it is usually at a natural point of narrowing, such as at the ileocecal valve. Increased viscosity of the feces may sometimes cause obstruction, especially in elderly persons and newborn infants. Hard, dry fecal masses may distend the sigmoid colon (fecal impaction). In infants with pancreatic disease, the meconium may be extremely viscid and sticky, causing chronic intestinal obstruction (meconium ileus). Rarely, a proximal segment of intestine projects into a more distal segment and blocks the lumen. This intussusception is most common in male infants, in whom it may occur without prior disease of the bowel. In adults, intussusception is usually secondary, as to a polypoid tumor of the mucosa.

Paralytic ileus may be due to gangrene of the bowel wall (as in ruptured gangrenous appendicitis or mesenteric thrombosis) or to other factors blocking nerve impulses. Injuries of the spinal cord, severe systemic infections such as pneumonia, metabolic disturbances such as hypokalemia or water intoxication, or inflammation of the peritoneum cause ileus.

Items 317-326

317. The causes of hepatocellular necrosis include all of the following **EXCEPT**:

    (A)   acetaminophen
    (B)   halothane
    (C)   hepatitis viruses
    (D)   phenobarbital
    (E)   yellow fever virus

318. A 6 year-old child had measles and was treated with aspirin. He developed Reye's syndrome. Pathologic changes in Reye's syndrome include all of the following **EXCEPT**:

    (A)   edema of the brain
    (B)   fatty change of the liver
    (C)   intrahepatic cholestasis
    (D)   lipid deposition in myocardial fibers
    (E)   lipid deposition in renal tubular epithelium

319. Several weeks after surgery during which he received a blood transfusion, a 45 year-old man developed jaundice, fever, nausea, and vomiting. Hepatitis was diagnosed. The virus most commonly transmitted during blood transfusion is

    (A)   hepatitis A
    (B)   hepatitis B
    (C)   hepatitis C
    (D)   hepatitis D (delta)
    (E)   human immunodeficiency virus (HIV)

320. A 45 year-old alcoholic went on a binge for 2 weeks. He was found comatose and in liver failure. His liver at autopsy showed hyaline Mallory bodies in the cytoplasm of hepatocytes. This finding is most typical of

   (A)   alcoholic hepatitis
   (B)   biliary cirrhosis
   (C)   hepatocarcinoma
   (D)   macronodular (postnecrotic) cirrhosis
   (E)   viral hepatitis

A 40 year-old man was brought to the emergency room when he vomited about 100 ml of blood. He had a swollen abdomen with a fluid wave. Spider angiomata were present on the skin of his chest. A photomicrograph of the underlying lesion in his liver is shown in Figure 5.2.

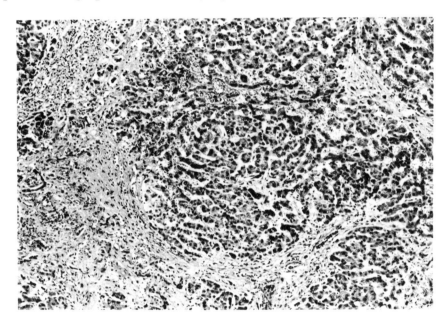

Figure 5.2

321. The likeliest diagnosis is

   (A)   biliary cirrhosis
   (B)   hepatocarcinoma
   (C)   macronodular cirrhosis
   (D)   micronodular cirrhosis
   (E)   viral hepatitis

322. A 55 year-old woman developed itching followed by jaundice. She was diagnosed as having primary biliary cirrhosis. All of the following are associated with biliary cirrhosis **EXCEPT**:

(A) chronic intrahepatic cholangitis
(B) hyaline (Mallory) bodies in hepatocytes
(C) markedly elevated serum alkaline phosphatase
(D) positive serum mitochondrial antibody test
(E) rheumatoid arthritis

323. Adenoma of the liver occurs in increased incidence in patients taking

(A) chlorpromazine
(B) cimetidine
(C) erythromycin
(D) oral contraceptives
(E) reserpine

324. The most common malignant neoplasm of the liver in the U.S. is

(A) carcinoid
(B) cholangiocarcinoma
(C) hepatocarcinoma
(D) Kaposi's sarcoma
(E) metastatic carcinoma

325. Hepatocarcinoma most commonly develops in a liver which is the site of

(A) aflatoxin toxicity
(B) cirrhosis
(C) Clonorchis sinensis infestation
(D) drug induced intrahepatic cholestasis
(E) hemochromatosis

326. Metabolic or endocrine abnormalities associated with hepatocarcinoma include all of the following **EXCEPT**:

(A) hypercalcemia due to parathormone secretion
(B) hypertension due to catecholamine secretion
(C) hypoglycemia
(D) polycythemia
(E) sexual precocity due to gonadotropin secretion

ANSWERS AND TUTORIAL ON ITEMS 317-326

The answers are: **317-D; 318-C; 319-C; 320-A; 321-D; 322-B; 323-D; 324-E; 325-B; 326-B**. Hepatic necrosis may be zonal, focal, or diffuse. Zonal necrosis is central in chronic passive congestion, midzonal in yellow fever, and peripheral in eclampsia and phosphorus poisoning early. In focal necrosis, small areas are affected without uniform distribution; it occurs in typhoid fever. Diffuse necrosis may be caused by drugs such as acetaminophen, isoniazid, and halothane; chemicals such as phosphorus and carbon tetrachloride; bacteria (Leptospira icterohaemorrhagiae), and the hepatitis viruses.

The age, sex, signs of portal hypertension with esophageal varices and ascites and the microscopic pattern of fibrosis about a single lobule without a central vein are all consistent with a diagnosis of micronodular cirrhosis in Item 321.

Encephalopathy with fatty changes in the liver and kidneys (Reye's syndrome) occurs in infants and children. The cause in unknown, but numerous cases have been associated with viral infections such as influenza. The use of aspirin has been implicated as a cause. Laboratory data include decreased blood and cerebrospinal fluid glucose levels. The mortality rate is about 75 percent. The liver is enlarged, firm, and yellow with severe fatty metamorphosis. The kidneys are increased in size, and there is lipid deposition in the cytoplasm of proximal convoluted tubular epithelium. The heart may be enlarged and pale. Extensive lipid droplet deposition is found in myocardial fibers. The brain is markedly edematous.

Viral hepatitis is caused by hepatitis viruses A, B, C, and D (delta). Hepatitis C (formerly non-A, non-B) is responsible for most cases transmitted via blood transfusions. Hepatitis virus A is transmitted by ingestion of fecally contaminated water or food. Hepatitis B virus is transmitted by plasma and blood transfusion, vaccines containing human serum, injections with contaminated needles and tattoo needles. Some cases of B virus hepatitis are transmitted by fecal contamination and by sexual contact. The delta agent can replicate only in the presence of hepatitis B surface antigen. The virus D can produce marked damage to hepatocytes.

The gross and microscopic appearance of the liver in viral hepatitis depends on the severity of the disease. In healthy carriers of HB_SAg, hepatocytes in liver biopsies have a ground-glass appearance. In nonfatal cases of acute hepatitis, biopsies show early degeneration of the parenchymal cells. The associated inflammatory reaction is mainly lymphocytic. In fulminating cases with early death, the liver is usually moderately reduced in size, very soft, dark reddish brown, and has a wrinkled capsule with massive destruction of liver cells, but the supporting reticulum is preserved.

Hepatic failure (cholemia) ensues when such a large part of the hepatic parenchyma has been destroyed that the organ is unable to carry on its functions. Hepatic coma results from the effects of hepatic failure on the brain. The encephalopathy of hepatic failure is due to a marked elevation of the serum ammonia. The elevated ammonia results from the decreased ability of the liver to produce urea, increased absorption of ammonia from the intestine secondary to gastrointestinal hemorrhage and a high protein diet, or increased ammonia retention due to the administration of diuretics.

Alcoholic hepatitis is a way station on the road to cirrhosis. It is characterized by the presence of alcoholic hyalin (Mallory bodies) especially in centrolobular hepatocytes. There is a neutrophilic inflammatory infiltrate, and fibroblastic proliferation lays down collagen around degenerating centrolobular cells. Central vein sclerosis also occurs. Later fibrous septa grow out as spurs toward the periphery of the lobule. These septa may be incomplete or may reach the portal triad as a bridge. Eventually, lobular architecture is destroyed by proliferation of bridges and bile ductules, parenchymal cell collapse, and nodular hepatocytic regeneration.

Micronodular (portal) cirrhosis is the most common form. Ethyl alcohol is the most important causative factor. Alcohol has direct and indirect toxic effects on the liver which play a role in the pathogenesis of portal cirrhosis. This type of cirrhosis is most common in men over 45. The liver may be enlarged early, weighing up to 5000 gm. or more, due to fatty metamorphosis, but later it becomes atrophic and may be reduced to one-half its normal size. Its surface is finely nodular, as is the cut surface. The nodules usually measure from 0.3 to 1.0 cm. in diameter. Groups of hepatic cells, usually several lobules, are surrounded by fibrous strands. The central veins disappear, and there is a severe disruption of the lobular architecture. Some degenerating hepatocytes contain a hyaline material which stains deeply with eosin (alcoholic hyalin).

Portal hypertension causes digestive symptoms, ascites, and splenomegaly. The portal hypertension is due to the compression of small venous radicles by fibrosis and by regenerating nodules of liver cells, and to an increase in the number and extent of arterioportal venous shunts. In an attempt to overcome the obstruction, various collateral channels develop, and about 85 percent of the portal venous blood bypasses the liver through collaterals. The collateral channels include dilatation of the anastomoses between the left coronary vein of the stomach and the esophageal veins. Esophageal varices may form, and rupture of such a varix is the most common cause of fatal hemorrhage in cirrhosis. Hemorrhoids develop because of the increased mesenteric venous pressure.

Biliary cirrhosis is rare. In most cases, it is secondary to chronic obstruction on the biliary passages (obstructive biliary cirrhosis). Chronic cholangitis and pericholangitis with intrahepatic cholestasis occurs in a number of patients with ulcerative colitis. In some of these cases, biliary cirrhosis develops. Primary biliary cirrhosis (PBC) is related to prolonged intrahepatic cholestasis. About 90 percent of the cases of PBC occur in women, usually between 40 and 60. Over 90 percent of the patients have positive serum mitochondrial antibody tests and elevated IgM levels. Association with hypersensitivity disorders such as lymphocytic thyroiditis, rheumatoid arthritis, and Sjögren's syndrome is common in patients with PBC.

Primary neoplasms of the liver are uncommon in the United States, although metastatic tumors to the liver are very frequent. Adenoma is a circumscribed, liver-colored mass consisting of well-differentiated hepatocytes without lobular organization. A number of cases of this rare neoplasm have developed in women taking oral contraceptives. Such adenomas tend to be large and undergo hemorrhage spontaneously or after mild trauma. Adenomas occasionally develop in children and adults on androgen therapy.

Hepatocarcinoma is the most common type of primary liver carcinoma, constituting about 80 percent of cases. A number of cases of hepatocarcinoma have been associated with marked hypoglycemia and a significant depression in blood sugar has been reported in about 30 percent of cases. The hypoglycemia is perhaps best explained by excessive use of glucose by and storage of glycogen in the neoplastic cells. Polycythemia (possibly due to erythropoietin production), hypercalcemia (due to parathormone secretion), and sexual precocity (due to elaboration of gonadotropin in children) have occurred in patients with hepatocarcinoma. Grossly, the liver is usually greatly enlarged weighing over 3000 gm. The neoplasms show three forms: multinodular, presenting varisized, circumscribed masses throughout the liver; massive, which is a large single mass; and diffuse. The neoplastic nodules are yellowish tan, often showing hemorrhagic or yellow necrotic foci. Microscopically, there are trabeculae or sheets of large atypical hepatocytes with numerous multinucleated neoplastic giant cells.

Hepatic cirrhosis, especially that due to chronic hepatitis B, is an associated finding in about 75 percent of hepatocarcinomas. About 8 percent of patients with cirrhosis develop primary liver carcinoma. Hepatitis B virus, aflatoxin, cycasin, and Clonorchis sinensis infestation have been implicated as causes of hepatocarcinoma. A few women using oral contraceptives have developed hepatocarcinoma.

Items 327-333

In Items 327-332, match each item with the type or types of gallstone to which it is most closely related.

        (A)   bilirubin pigment gallstones
        (B)   cholesterol gallstones
        (C)   both
        (D)   neither

327.   diabetes mellitus

328.   estrogen therapy

329.   hemolytic anemia

330.   hyperparathyroidism

331.   ileal resection

332.   infection of gallbladder by bacteria producing ß-glucuronidase

333. The complications of gallstones include all of the following **EXCEPT**:

   (A)   adenocarcinoma of ampulla of Vater
   (B)   acute intrahepatic cholangitis
   (C)   acute pancreatitis
   (D)   gangrenous cholecystitis
   (E)   intestinal obstruction

ANSWERS AND TUTORIAL ON ITEMS 327-333

The answers are: **327-B; 328-B; 329-A; 330-D; 331-B; 332-A; 333-A**. Cholelithiasis is the formation of calculi (gallstones) in the gallbladder. Stones are about 2.5 times as frequent in females as in males and are especially frequent in women who have borne children, in diabetics, and in the obese. An increased incidence of cholesterol gallstones has been reported in women taking oral contraceptives. Cholesterol gallstones are also increased in frequency in both women and men on estrogen therapy. Patients using clofibrate have an increased incidence of cholesterol stones because of increased cholesterol levels in bile. Individuals who have had an ileal resection or bypass operation are prone to develop cholesterol stones because of decreased bile acid absorption and depletion of the bile acid pool in the liver. The incidence of cholesterol stones is also increased in Crohn's disease.

   About 10 percent of all gallstones are composed of pure cholesterol. Such a stone is usually about 1 to 2 cm. in diameter, light weight, and rounded. Often only one stone is present. The bile salts and lecithin are essential for the formation of micelles which hold cholesterol in solution in bile. Cholesterol stone formation may result from loss of stability in this micellar solution in the liver or the gallbladder. Such instability may be due to a relative increase in cholesterol or decrease in bile salt or lecithin concentration in the bile. There is no direct relationship between hypercholesterolemia and the development of a cholesterol gallstone. About 10 percent of all gallstones are composed of bile pigment. They are usually 2 to 5 mm. in diameter, multiple, faceted, dark green to black, and smooth; they crumble easily on pressure and are homogeneous and putty-like. This type of stone is commonly found in the gallbladder in long-standing cases of hemolytic anemia. Pigment stones are also common in infected bile because of the release of ß-glucuronidase by bacteria. This enzyme converts water soluble conjugated bilirubin to the insoluble unconjugated form, increasing the likelihood of calcium bilirubinate stone formation. Mixed and combined stones together make up about 80 percent of all gallstones. They contain both cholesterol and bile pigment, often in concentric layers of nearly pure substance, together with calcium carbonate and calcium bilirubinate.

   The complications of gallstones include gangrenous cholecystitis by pressure on the mucosa and blood vessels in an acutely inflamed gallbladder; cholangitis by blocking the major biliary ducts and allowing bacteria to ascend into the liver; obstructive jaundice by blocking the common duct; acute pancreatitis by blocking the ampulla of Vater or a major pancreatic duct; and intestinal obstruction at the ileocecal valve (gallstone ileus).

334. A 50 year-old man attended a banquet where he had several drinks and a heavy meal. A few hours later he had severe upper abdominal pain and vomiting. He went into shock. The most likely diagnosis is

   (A)   acute cholecystitis
   (B)   acute gastroenteritis
   (C)   acute pancreatitis
   (D)   intussusception
   (E)   perforated duodenal ulcer

335. Typical laboratory findings in acute hemorrhagic pancreatitis include all of the following **EXCEPT**:

   (A)   decreased serum calcium
   (B)   increased serum amylase
   (C)   increased serum ammonia
   (D)   increased hematocrit
   (E)   increased serum lipase

336. An increased incidence of acute pancreatitis is associated with all of the following **EXCEPT**:

   (A)   alcoholism
   (B)   cholelithiasis
   (C)   chlorothiazide therapy
   (D)   hyperparathyroidism
   (E)   hypertension

In Items 337-342, match each item with the heading with which it is most closely related.

   (A)   carcinoma of head of pancreas
   (B)   micronodular cirrhosis of liver
   (C)   both
   (D)   neither

337. decreased serum albumin

338. elevated serum cholesterol

339. elevated serum bilirubin

340. greatly elevated serum alkaline phosphatase

341. elevated serum uric acid

342. prolonged prothrombin time

343. All of the following are features of pancreatic carcinoma **EXCEPT**:

   (A) carcinoembryonic antigen test is often positive
   (B) most cases develop in the head of the pancreas
   (C) obstructive jaundice may be a presenting sign
   (D) phlebothrombosis tends to occur
   (E) there is a significant association with cystic fibrosis of the pancreas

ANSWERS AND TUTORIAL ON ITEMS 334-343

The answers are: **334-C; 335-C; 336-E; 337-B; 338-A; 339-C; 340-A; 341-D; 342-C; 343-E**. Acute pancreatitis is seen chiefly in males after age 40 and often associated with obesity and alcoholism. In about 50 percent of the cases, gallstones are also present. Pancreatitis occurs in about 10 percent of cases of hyperparathyroidism. In some cases, calculi resulting from the hypercalcemia of hyperparathyroidism develop in pancreatic ducts and lead to obstruction and inflammation. A few cases of pancreatitis have occurred in patients taking chlorothiazide diuretics.

With the release of pancreatic enzymes into the interstitial tissue of the pancreas, a series of related biochemical and pathologic changes occur. The enzymes begin the digestion of the interstitial tissue. Fat necrosis develops in the pancreas and peripancreatic tissues, and often in the mesentery and omentum as well. Amylase and lipase are absorbed into the blood where they may appear in very high levels for a few days. In the foci of fat necrosis, the neutral fats are split into fatty acids and glycerol. The fatty acids unite with calcium from the blood to produce calcium soaps. The level of the serum calcium is lowered by this transfer to the tissues, in some cases in quantities sufficient to cause tetany. Shock and hemoconcentration lead to an increased hematocrit.

Carcinoma of the pancreas is more frequent in men than women and occurs usually in the sixth and seventh decades. In about 90 percent of cases, the carcinoembryonic antigen test is positive. A migratory phlebothrombosis is associated in about one-third of the cases (Trousseau's syndrome). About 75 percent of pancreatic carcinomas appear in the head. The neoplasm is a poorly defined, hard, nodular, light tan mass measuring up to 10 cm. in diameter within the pancreas. Most of the neoplasms are adenocarcinomas derived from duct epithelium, showing irregular spaces lined by one or more layers of atypical cylindrical epithelium. A dense fibrous stroma is often present. Less common is the acinar cell carcinoma. Metastases are most common to the periaortic and mesenteric lymph nodes, peritoneum, liver, and lungs.

Items 337-342 deal with the differentiation of obstructive jaundice (carcinoma of head of pancreas) and hepatogenous jaundice (micronodular cirrhosis). Elevated serum bilirubin occurs in both, mainly conjugated in obstruction and mixed in liver cell damage. Elevated cholesterol and markedly increased alkaline phosphatase occur with obstruction to the outflow of bile in which both are excreted. Albumin is decreased with hepatocellular loss because of decreased synthesis. The prothrombin time is lengthened in both - because of decreased synthesis from vitamin K in hepatic damage and because of failure of absorption of fat solvent soluble vitamin K with the absence of bile in the small intestine due to bile duct obstruction.

CHAPTER VI

URINARY SYSTEM PATHOLOGY

Items 344-352

A 50 year-old man was found to have hypertension, proteinuria, azotemia, and anemia. KUB X-ray films demonstrated greatly enlarged kidney shadows. The kidneys were removed in preparation for a transplant. A photograph of the gross kidney specimens is shown in Figure 6.1.

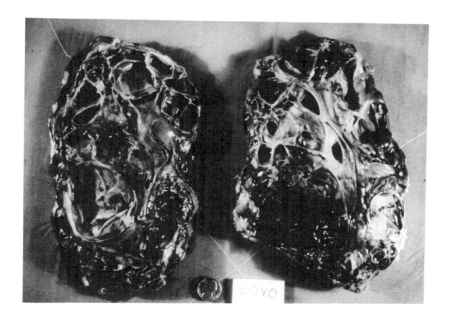

Figure 6.1

344. The likeliest diagnosis is

    (A) bilateral renal adenocarcinoma
    (B) bilateral hydronephrosis
    (C) hereditary nephritis (Alport's syndrome)
    (D) acquired cysts of kidneys
    (E) polycystic kidneys

345. Immune complex deposition in a "lumpy, bumpy" pattern along glomerular basement membranes is found in all of the following **EXCEPT**:

    (A)   acute proliferative glomerulonephritis
    (B)   dense deposit glomerulonephritis
    (C)   lupus nephritis
    (D)   membranous glomerulonephropathy
    (E)   minimal change disease

346. A 10 year-old boy developed a pharyngitis due to ß-hemolytic streptococci. It subsided after a few days of penicillin therapy. Two weeks later his eyelids became puffy, and he had fever, elevated blood pressure, and gross hematuria. The likeliest diagnosis is

    (A)   acute proliferative glomerulonephritis
    (B)   antiglomerular basement membrane disease
    (C)   membranous glomerulonephropathy
    (D)   minimal change disease
    (E)   rapidly progressive glomerulonephritis

347. A 35 year-old man developed hematuria, proteinuria, mounting azotemia, and hypertension. A renal biopsy confirmed the diagnosis of rapidly progressive glomerulonephritis. The most characteristic microscopic finding in this condition is

    (A)   epithelial crescents within glomeruli
    (B)   hyalinization of numerous glomeruli
    (C)   hyalinization of walls of afferent arterioles
    (D)   proliferation of glomerular tuft and mesangial cells
    (E)   uniform thickening of glomerular basement membranes

348. A 25 year-old man developed hematuria and hemoptysis. Immunofluorescent studies on a renal biopsy demonstrated linear immune globulin deposits along glomerular basement membranes. The most likely diagnosis is

    (A)   acute proliferative glomerulonephritis
    (B)   diabetic glomerulosclerosis
    (C)   Goodpasture's syndrome
    (D)   lupus nephritis
    (E)   membranous glomerulonephropathy

349. An 8 year-old girl was found to have the nephrotic syndrome. The commonest cause of this disorder in children is

   (A)   acute proliferative glomerulonephritis
   (B)   membranous glomerulonephropathy
   (C)   minimal change glomerulonephropathy
   (D)   nephroblastoma (Wilms' tumor)
   (E)   rapidly progressive glomerulonephritis

350. Characteristic features of the nephrotic syndrome include all of the following **EXCEPT**:

   (A)   edema
   (B)   hypercholesterolemia
   (C)   hypoalbuminemia
   (D)   hypokalemia
   (E)   proteinuria

351. A 30 year-old man developed edema, proteinuria, hypoproteinemia, and hypercholesterolemia. A renal biopsy showed uniform thickening of glomerular basement membranes. Immunofluorescence revealed lumpy deposits of immune globulins and complement along the basement membranes. The diagnosis of membranous glomerulonephropathy was made. This condition may be secondary to all of the following **EXCEPT**:

   (A)   amyloidosis
   (B)   hepatitis B
   (C)   lupus erythematosus
   (D)   malignant neoplasm
   (E)   renal vein thrombosis

352. A patient with chronic glomerulonephritis developed renal failure. Laboratory findings which would be expected in this patient include all of the following **EXCEPT**:

   (A)   anemia
   (B)   elevated serum ammonia
   (C)   elevated serum calcium
   (D)   elevated serum creatinine
   (E)   hyposthenuria

ANSWERS AND TUTORIAL ON ITEMS 344-352

The answers are: **344-E; 345-E; 346-A; 347-A; 348-C; 349-C; 350-D; 351-A; 352-C**.

> In Item 344, this is the so-called adult type of polycystic kidneys which is due to a developmental defect but does not become apparent until middle age.
>
> A "lumpy, bumpy" pattern of deposition is due to circulating immune complexes which appear to be trapped on the endothelial side, within, or on the epithelial side of the glomerular basement membrane. It occurs in the disorders listed in Item 345, except minimal change disease.
>
> Item 346 gives a classical history for the development of acute poststreptococcal glomerulonephritis. Epithelial crescents are the typical microscopic feature of rapidly progressive glomerulonephritis.
>
> The combination of hematuria and hemoptysis in Item 348 in a young man is characteristic of Goodpasture's syndrome in which autoantibodies develop against the glomerular and pulmonary capillary basement membranes.
>
> The nephrotic syndrome occurs most often in minimal change disease (Item 349) in children and in membranous glomerulonephropathy in adults (Item 351).

Polycystic kidneys of the adult is transmitted as an autosomal dominant. The kidneys are enlarged, weighing up to 1750 gm. each. At birth the involvement is usually microcystic. In adults, the cysts may be very large. They are filled with clear to straw-colored watery fluid or with dark brown or blue fluid due to hemorrhage. Microscopically varying numbers of normal or compressed, functional nephrons are present between cysts. Hepatic cysts are common, and a berry aneurysm of an artery of the circle of Willis is found in about 15 percent of cases of adult polycystic kidneys.

There are two immune mechanisms of glomerular injury, (1) the deposition of circulating immune complexes or (2) of antiglomerular basement membrane antibodies. In immune complex disease, non-glomerular soluble antigen-antibody complexes are formed in the presence of an antigen excess. The antigen may be exogenous, as in ß-hemolytic streptococcal infections; or it may be endogenous, as in lupus erythematosus. Immune complexes of optimum size (molecular weight about 1 million) are trapped along the glomerular basement membrane during filtration. The complexes fix complement, and the anaphylotoxins C'3a and C'5a activate an acute inflammatory response. Glomerular basement membrane injury is caused by the release of lysosomal enzymes from PMNs and the lytic effect of C'5-9. Vasoactive amines released from degranulated mast cells and platelets increase membrane permeability. The immune complexes and complement occur along the glomerular basement membrane an a granular "lumpy, bumpy" pattern.

In antiglomerular basement membrane disease (AGBMD), which occurs much less often than immune complex disease, antibodies are produced against the antigen on glomerular basement membrane. The antigen may be protein constituent of the basement membrane (autoimmune AGBMD) or a foreign antigen fixed to the membrane. The antigen-antibody complexes form a linear pattern along the endothelial side of the glomerular basement membrane. The mechanisms of injury is the same as in immune complex disease. This pattern occurs in Goodpasture's syndrome.

Acute proliferative (postinfectious) glomerulonephritis is a generalized inflammation of the glomeruli with secondary tubular, interstitial, and vascular changes. In about 90 percent of patients with acute glomerulonephritis, there is an associated Group A, type 12 ß-hemolytic streptococcal infection, but occasional cases are associated with types 4, 1, 25, and 49. Usually the preceding infection is in the form of streptococcal pharyngitis or tonsillitis. Acute proliferative glomerulonephritis typically follows the antecedent infection after an interval of about 2 weeks. Most cases occur in the 5 to 20 age group. There is no correlation between the occurrence of acute rheumatic carditis and poststreptococcal glomerulonephritis.

In acute glomerulonephritis the kidneys are swollen, red, and smooth, with tense capsules which strip easily. The glomeruli are enlarged, and there is marked endothelial and mesangial cell proliferation. Many PMNs are present intra- and extravascularly. RBCs may be found in Bowman's spaces. Immunofluorescence reveals the presence of immune globulin G (IgG) and complement along the glomerular basement membranes in a lumpy, bumpy pattern characteristic of immune complex glomerulonephritis.

Proliferative glomerulonephritis with crescents (rapidly progressive glomerulonephritis) is usually idiopathic but may occur in poststreptococcal GN, Goodpasture's syndrome, lupus erythematosus, or Henoch-Schönlein purpura. The kidneys are large, pale and soft with widespread glomerular epithelial crescent formation due to proliferation of Bowman's capsular epithelium. The epithelial cells become fusiform. Collagen may be laid down in the crescents. The escape of fibrinogen through the damaged glomerular basement membrane with the formation of fibrin in the glomerular space is the stimulus for epithelial crescent formation.

Goodpasture's syndrome is an autoimmune disorder in which antiglomerular basement membrane antibodies are formed. This results in the deposition of immune globulin G and complement in a uniform linear pattern along the glomerular basement membranes. IgG and complement are also deposited along alveolar septa in the lungs, because the anti-GBM antibodies cross-react with alveolar basement membranes. In Goodpasture's syndrome, the lungs are heavy, often weighing up to 2000 gm. together. There is an acute necrotizing alveolitis with hemorrhage into the alveolar spaces. Early the kidneys show an acute proliferative glomerulonephritis, which changes into rapidly progressive glomerulonephritis with epithelial crescent formation in glomeruli.

Minimal change glomerulonephropathy, which occurs in males more often than in females, is the commonest cause of nephrotic syndrome in children. The nephrotic syndrome consists of massive proteinuria; hypoalbuminemia due to the urinary loss; widespread edema due to decreased plasma osmotic pressure; and hyperlipidemia, probably due to increased hepatic lipoprotein synthesis. The cause of minimal change disease is unknown. The kidneys are slightly enlarged and pale or yellow due to tubular lipids. The glomeruli have diffuse obliteration of the epithelial foot processes.

Membranous glomerulonephropathy is an immune complex disease of unknown cause. It usually occurs in young and middle-aged adults, being more common in males than in females. Membranous glomerulonephropathy is often primary but also occurs in cases of hepatitis B, lupus erythematosus, syphilis, sarcoidosis, malaria, renal vein thrombosis, and gold therapy. In patients over 50 years of age, membranous glomerulonephropathy is significantly associated with coexistent malignant neoplasm. The kidneys are slight to moderately enlarged, soft, and pale, mottled yellowish-red. The glomeruli show uniform thickening of the basement

143

membrane and even some proliferation of endothelial cells. Electron microscopy shows projections like the teeth of a comb on the epithelial side of the basement membrane; dense subepithelial deposits; and epithelial cell foot process fusion. There are lumpy deposits of IgG, IgM, and complement along the basement membrane.

Chronic glomerulonephritis is the slowly progressive end stage of proliferative or membranous glomerulonephritis. It may follow the active stage directly or appear after months or years. About half the cases develop without previously recognized renal disease. Hypertension increases steadily with progression of the disease. Renal findings include a loss of ability to concentrate urine with the development of a fixed specific gravity near 1.010 (hyposthenuria). The blood findings include elevated blood urea nitrogen (BUN), uric acid, creatinine, phosphate, chloride, and ammonia levels. The calcium level falls due to phosphate retention. Anemia may be pronounced late. This stage may last for years, terminating in uremia and death. The kidneys are symmetrically shriveled and firm, with tightly bound capsules which decorticate on stripping. The external surfaces are irregularly granular and pitted. The cortices are narrowed. Many glomeruli are hyalinized. or replaced by interstitial fibrous tissue infiltrated by lymphocytes.

Items 353-360

353.   The typical microscopic feature of toxic nephrosis is

      (A)   degeneration of proximal convoluted tubular epithelium
      (B)   degeneration of distal convoluted tubular epithelium
      (C)   interstitial edema and lymphocytic infiltration
      (D)   necrotizing papillitis
      (E)   tubulorrhexis (focal rupture of tubular basement membranes)

354.   The causes of hypoxic nephrosis include all of the following **EXCEPT**:

      (A)   excessive postpartum hemorrhage
      (B)   hemolytic transfusion reaction
      (C)   gram-negative septicemia
      (D)   hypokalemia
      (E)   trauma to muscles

355.   The most characteristic feature in a patient with acute tubular necrosis is

      (A)   hematuria
      (B)   hyposthenuria
      (C)   oliguria
      (D)   proteinuria
      (E)   pyuria

356. A 50 year-old woman was found on routine physical examination to have a blood pressure of 160/100. She was diagnosed as having essential hypertension. The most characteristic microscopic finding in a renal biopsy in essential hypertension is

    (A) epithelial crescents within glomeruli
    (B) hyalinization of numerous glomeruli
    (C) hyalinization of the walls of afferent arterioles
    (D) interstitial hemorrhage
    (E) interstitial fibrosis and lymphocytic infiltration

357. Endocrine disorders associated with the development of secondary hypertension include all of the following **EXCEPT**:

    (A) Conn's syndrome (aldosterone producing adrenal adenoma)
    (B) Cushing's syndrome
    (C) diabetes mellitus
    (D) pheochromocytoma
    (E) primary hyperthyroidism

358. Renal findings in cases of multiple myeloma include all of the following **EXCEPT**:

    (A) amyloid deposition in glomeruli and arterioles
    (B) Bence-Jones protein casts in tubules
    (C) metastatic calcification of tubules
    (D) necrotizing papillitis
    (E) plasma cell infiltration of interstitium

359. In diabetes mellitus renal lesions include all of the following **EXCEPT**:

    (A) acute pyelonephritis
    (B) glycogen deposition in tubular epithelium
    (C) necrotizing papillitis
    (D) nephrolithiasis
    (E) nodular glomerulosclerosis

360. The drug which causes renal papillary necrosis is

    (A) acetophenetidin
    (B) gentamicin
    (C) gold
    (D) methicillin
    (E) methoxyflurane

ANSWERS AND TUTORIAL ON ITEMS 353-360

The answers are: **353A; 354-D; 355-C; 356-C; 357-E; 358-D; 359-D; 360-A.**

Acute tubular necrosis includes all damage to renal tubules whether it is caused directly by chemical or drugs (toxic nephrosis) or indirectly by a reduction in blood supply or precipitation of hemoglobin or myoglobin (hypoxic nephrosis). Oliguria or anuria is the most common clinical feature of all types of acute tubular necrosis. Degeneration of proximal convoluted tubular epithelium is typical in toxic nephrosis. In hypoxic nephrosis, more distal portions of the convoluted tubules are involved. Shock and hemolytic reactions are the basis for most cases of hypoxic nephrosis.

Hypertension is a complex subject, but the most usual microscopic finding in the kidneys is a simple one - hyalinization of afferent arterioles of glomeruli. This is a result of the increased pressure.

The renal findings in multiple myeloma and diabetes mellitus are protean and involve glomeruli, tubules, blood vessels, and interstitium.

Among the chemical agents which cause toxic nephrosis are mercuric chloride, carbon tetrachloride, and ethylene glycol. Oliguria or anuria may be partly due to tubular blockage and/or reabsorption of the glomerular filtrate. After a few weeks, if the patient survives, diuresis with dilute urine ensues. The kidneys are markedly swollen. The renal capsule is tense, stripping easily to reveal a smooth pale red or yellow surface. In the proximal convoluted tubules, necrosis extends down to but does not include the basement membrane.

Hypoxic (ischemic) nephrosis may occur in shock, burns, septicemia, crush syndrome, heat stroke, hemolytic transfusion reactions, and postoperatively. Shock with decreased renal cortical blood flow is most likely the basic cause. The renal insufficiency is probably due to blockage of the tubules by pigment casts and the swelling of the epithelial cells and vasoconstrictive renal ischemia due to shock. The kidneys are enlarged, flabby, and pale. Degenerative changes occur in the epithelium of the distal convoluted tubules. The necrosis extends down to and produces focal rupture of the tubular basement membrane (tubulorrhexis). Hemoglobin or myoglobin casts appear mainly in the distal convoluted and collecting tubules.

A patient is hypertensive if the systolic blood pressure is persistently above 140 mm of Hg. or the diastolic blood pressure is above 90 mm. In about 90 percent of the cases of hypertensive cardiovascular disease, no definite cause for hypertension can be identified (primary or essential hypertension).

In the remaining 10 percent of the cases of hypertension, some organic or functional disorder is believed to account for the elevation of blood pressure. These include: increased intracranial pressure; spinal cord lesions; diseases of the urinary tract, including polycystic kidneys, glomerulonephritis, pyelonephritis, diabetic glomerulosclerosis, scleroderma, polyarteritis nodosa, renin-secreting tumor, and obstruction of blood flow in one renal artery; endocrine disturbances, particularly lesions of the adrenal gland such as pheochromocytoma, those associated with increased secretion of aldosterone, or Cushing's syndrome; toxemia of pregnancy; and coarctation of the aorta.

Arteriolonephrosclerosis is the most constant pathologic finding in benign essential hypertension. The kidneys become moderately or markedly atrophic due to cortical narrowing.

The essential lesion is a marked sclerosis in the afferent arterioles just proximal to the glomerular tuft. Other small arteries and arterioles show hyaline thickening. The lumina are narrowed or even obliterated. The hyalin is made up of compact fine granules and appears to arise by excessive filtration of plasma proteins into the arterioles.

Myeloma nephrosis occurs in some cases of multiple myeloma. Bence-Jones protein appears in the urine in patients and severe renal damage due to precipitation of the protein in the tubules. The kidneys are slightly or markedly reduced in size. The cut surfaces are pale and waxy. Many distal convoluted tubules are blocked by highly eosinophilic Bence-Jones protein casts. The adjacent tubular epithelium shows a syncytium interpreted as a multinucleated foreign body giant cell reaction. Other renal lesions associated with multiple myeloma include metastatic calcification in the tubules from destructive bone lesions, occasional plasma cell infiltration in the interstitial tissue, and amyloid deposits in glomeruli and arterioles.

Diabetic glomerulosclerosis is one of the most distinctive renal lesions in diabetes mellitus. The kidneys are usually slightly larger than normal and are not diagnostic grossly. In the nodular type, there are round, hyaline masses in the mesangium of glomeruli which represent basement membrane material. In the diffuse type, there is a generalized thickening of the glomerular basement membranes due to accumulation of epithelial basal lamina material. The diffuse and nodular forms of diabetic glomerulosclerosis frequently occur together. Other renal lesions in diabetes mellitus include necrotizing papillitis and both fatty changes and the accumulation of glycogen in the convoluted tubular epithelium. Arteriolonephrosclerosis is common in diabetics in association with hypertension. Distinctive of diabetes is hyaline thickening of the efferent as well as the afferent arterioles. Acute and chronic pyelonephritis occur fairly frequently in diabetics. The necrotizing papillitis in diabetes is usually fulminant and associated with a severe ascending urinary tract infection. Renal papillary necrosis due to acetophenetidin is a gradual process with slow loss of renal function.

361. A 10 year-old boy with osteomyelitis began to have pain in both flanks and burning on urination. He had pus and bacteria in his urine and was diagnosed as having acute hematogenous pyelonephritis. The commonest causative organism for this condition is

    (A) Aerobacter aerogenes
    (B) Escherichia coli
    (C) Proteus vulgaris
    (D) Staphylococcus aureus
    (E) Streptococcus faecalis

362. A 35 year-old mother of 6 children with a history of hypertension died of renal failure. At autopsy the kidneys were atrophic and unequal in size (right 80 gm., left 100 gm.), had wide U-shaped scars on their surfaces, and slightly dilated pelves and calyces with scarring of their walls. The cut surfaces were grossly fibrotic. The likeliest diagnosis is

    (A) arteriolonephrosclerosis
    (B) chronic glomerulonephritis
    (C) chronic pyelonephritis
    (D) hereditary nephritis
    (E) stenosis of one renal artery

363. Glitter cells are most characteristic in the urine in cases of

    (A) acute proliferative glomerulonephritis
    (B) acute pyelonephritis
    (C) diabetic glomerulosclerosis
    (D) membranous glomerulonephritis
    (E) minimal change glomerulonephropathy

364. Predisposing factors for the development of renal calculi include all of the following **EXCEPT**:

    (A) dehydration
    (B) hypercholesterolemia
    (C) hyperparathyroidism
    (D) hypervitaminosis D
    (E) urinary tract infection

A 40 year-old man was found to have an enlarged nonfunctional kidney. It was surgically removed. A photograph of the gross specimen is shown in Figure 6.2.

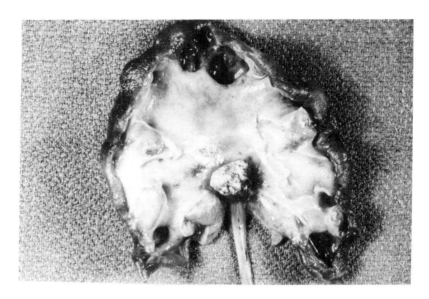

Figure 6.2

365.   In this specimen, all of the following pathologic changes are likely to be present **EXCEPT**:

(A)   calculus formation
(B)   cortical atrophy
(C)   chronic pyelonephritis
(D)   hydronephrosis
(E)   infarction

366.   The chemical composition of renal calculi may be any of the following **EXCEPT**:

(A)   calcium carbonate
(B)   calcium oxalate
(C)   calcium oxalate and phosphate
(D)   magnesium and ammonium phosphate
(E)   uric acid

A 50 year-old man developed hematuria. He was found to have a large neoplasm in his right kidney, which was surgically removed. A photograph of the gross specimen is shown in Figure 6.3.

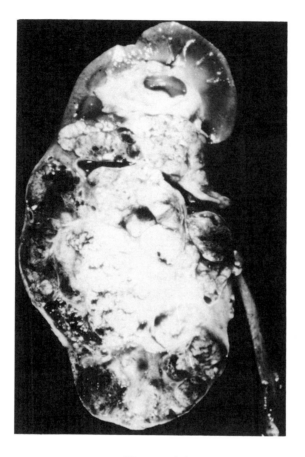

Figure 6.3

367. The neoplasm shown in the photograph arises from

    (A)   adrenal cortical rests
    (B)   glomerular epithelium
    (C)   metanephrogenic blastema
    (D)   proximal convoluted tubular epithelium
    (E)   collecting tubular epithelium

368. An intravenous pyelogram demonstrated that a patient had bilateral hydronephrosis and hydroureter. Causes of bilateral urinary obstruction may include all of the following **EXCEPT**:

(A) adenocarcinoma of prostate gland
(B) periureteral fibrosis
(C) renal papillary necrosis due to analgesics
(D) stage IV carcinoma of the cervix
(E) urethral stricture

369. The causes of ureteral obstruction include all of the following **EXCEPT**:

(A) acute ureteritis
(B) lower polar renal artery
(C) papillary carcinoma of ureter
(D) renal calculus
(E) ureteral stricture

370. A 2 year-old child was found to have a large mass arising from the right kidney. The most frequent malignant renal neoplasm in children is

(A) adenocarcinoma
(B) lymphoma
(C) nephroblastoma (Wilms' tumor)
(D) neuroblastoma
(E) papillary carcinoma

371. Concerning nephroblastoma, all of the following statements are true **EXCEPT**:

(A) about 10 percent of cases are bilateral
(B) it originates from cells of the metanephrogenic blastema
(C) it is a golden yellow mass with focal hemorrhage and necrosis
(D) some patients have a deletion in a short arm of chromosome 11
(E) there is a significant association with aniridia

372. A 60 year-old man had dysuria and hematuria. On cystoscopy he was found to have a papillary transitional cell carcinoma of the urinary bladder. Causative factors in the development of bladder cancer include all of the following **EXCEPT**:

(A) aniline dyes
(B) ß-naphthylamine
(C) heavy cigarette smoking
(D) salicylates
(E) schistosomiasis of the bladder

373. Pathologic changes in patients dying of uremia include all of the following **EXCEPT**:

(A) anemia due to failure of erythropoietin production
(B) edema of the brain
(C) fibrinous pericarditis
(D) multiple renal cysts in those on long term dialysis
(E) phlebothrombosis

ANSWERS AND TUTORIAL ON ITEMS 361-373

The answers are: **361-D; 362-C; 363-B; 364-B; 365-E; 366-A; 367-D; 368-C; 369-A; 370-C; 371-C; 372-D; 373-E**.

Bacterial infections of the kidneys may be ascending (typically from Escherichia coli) (90%) or hematogenous (typically from Staphylococcus aureus) (10%). Glitter cells are neutrophils found in the urine showing Brownian movement of the cytoplasmic granules. Their presence in the urine is highly suggestive of the diagnosis of pyelonephritis.

It is often difficult to determine the underlying cause of chronically scarred kidneys. In arteriolonephrosclerosis and chronic glomerulonephritis, both kidneys are affected equally and so are symmetrically scarred. In chronic pyelonephritis, involvement is often uneven, and the pelves and calyces show signs of old infection. In renal artery stenosis, the ipsilateral kidney is atrophic while the contralateral one is compensatorily large.

Urinary calculi are for the most part due to hypercalciuria and have no relation to cholesterol metabolism. Any factor that tends to concentrate calcium in the urine predisposes to stone formation.

Bilateral renal obstruction must involve both ureters, the bladder neck, or the urethra. Ureteral obstruction may be caused by intrinsic or extrinsic narrowing or obliteration of the lumen.

Adenocarcinoma of the kidney arises from proximal convoluted tubular epithelium, and the nephroblastoma from the metanephrogenic blastema. Wilms' tumor is sometimes part of a multiple developmental defect complex.

Pyelonephritis denotes an infection of the kidney and renal pelvis. In pyelonephritis, the infecting organism may reach the kidneys either hematogenously or urogenously, the latter via the ureteral lumen as an ascending infection. Some type of obstruction to the normal outflow or urine is usually present, especially in the ascending types. There is a uniformly higher evidence of urinary tract infection in females than males due to the shortness of the female urethra and ureteral kinking and compression during pregnancy.

Acute pyelonephritis may be unilateral or bilateral. The involved kidney is enlarged and hyperemic. Yellow abscesses of various sizes are found in the medulla. These radiate up into the cortex. The pelvic mucosa is red and edematous, and the calyces and pelvis contain pus. Interstitial tissue and sometimes tubules are infiltrated with PMNs.

Cases of chronic pyelonephritis often show progressive renal failure. Bacteria are seldom found in the renal parenchyma except in those cases in which demonstrable urinary obstruction is present. The kidneys are small, often weighing less than 100 gm. each. Points which tend to differentiate the contracted kidneys of chronic pyelonephritis from those of arteriolonephrosclerosis and chronic glomerulonephritis grossly are inequality in the size and weight of the kidneys, the presence of wide U-shaped depressions on the external surfaces, the presence of dilated calyces and pelves indicating urinary obstruction, and grayish white scarring of the pelvic and calycine submucosa. Microscopically there are clusters of hyalinized glomeruli adjacent to foci of dilated tubules containing eosinophilic colloid casts (thyroidization of the kidney), periglomerular fibrosis, interstitial fibrosis with a moderate to marked interstitial infiltration with lymphocytes, plasmacytes, and macrophages, and hyaline thickening of the walls of arterioles and small arteries.

Urolithiasis is the formation of calculi (stones) within the urinary tract. They most often begin in the renal calyces and pelvis, sometimes later being passed into the ureter or bladder. Men have a higher incidence of renal calculi than women.

An important primary etiologic factor is supersaturation of the urine with crystalline material. Most commonly this is in the form of calcium salts, the hypercalciuria being idiopathic or due to primary or secondary hyperparathyroidism, extensive bone demineralization, hypervitaminosis D, or an excessive intake of milk and alkalis. Calculi develop particularly when there is prolonged recumbent bed rest with osteoporosis or when there is dehydration. Stones due to supersaturation are typically bilateral and tend to recur.

Calcium oxalate stones make up about one-third of all urinary calculi. They occur in acid urine, are dark brown, oval, extremely hard and rough, and usually measure less than 1 cm. Roughly 40 percent of urinary calculi consist of calcium oxalate combined with calcium phosphate. This stone occurs mainly in alkaline urine and is due to hypercalciuria with secondary urinary tract infection. About 20 percent of calculi are magnesium and ammonium phosphate stones. These usually form in alkaline urine and in association with infection. They often encrust on a foreign body or neoplasm in the urinary bladder. They may become very large as staghorn calculi in the kidneys. Uric acid stones form in some cases of gout.

Obstruction of the urinary tract may occur anywhere from the renal tubules to the urethral meatus. Pelvic obstruction is usually partial and is caused by a large renal calculus or pelvic neoplasm. Ureteral obstruction may be due to intraluminal blockage (calculus, primary neoplasm); external pressure (lower polar renal artery; periureteral fibrosis; secondary neoplasm, especially carcinoma of the cervix by extension to one or both ureters; congenital or acquired stricture); kinking (pregnancy). Pelvic and ureteral obstruction are usually chronic and partial and may be constant or intermittent. Most cases are unilateral. Vesical obstruction is caused by a large calculus and by primary or secondary neoplasm, especially in the trigone. Except for neoplasm about a single ureteral orifice, obstruction in the bladder affects both ureters and kidneys. Bladder neck obstruction is an important cause of urinary blockage in children. Urethral obstruction is caused by compression due to hyperplasia or carcinoma of the prostate, which also constricts the bladder neck; gonorrheal stricture; urethral neoplasms; and congenital anomalies.

Adenocarcinoma of the kidney constitutes about 85 percent of malignant renal neoplasms. It occurs in men twice as often as in women, and develops after age 40 in 90 percent of the cases. The cause is unknown. In cases of hereditary renal adenocarcinoma, there is a balanced reciprocal translocation between chromosome 3 and 8. The neoplasm arises from renal tubular epithelium and is probably related to the renal adenoma. Grossly renal adenocarcinoma is typically a large, roughly spherical, partially encapsulated, golden yellow mass. The cut surface shows extensive foci of necrosis and hemorrhage. The neoplasm occurs most commonly at the upper pole and compresses the adjacent renal parenchyma. Microscopically the tumor is most frequently composed of clusters of large cells with a clear cytoplasm. The cells have a high lipid content, which gives the neoplasm its yellow color. Metastases are usually the result of invasion of the renal vein. Sometimes the neoplasm grows into the inferior vena cava, and even into the right atrium. Metastases to the lungs are sometimes discrete, spherical "cannon ball" masses.

Nephroblastoma (Wilms' tumor) is a congenital malignant neoplasm. It makes up about 5 percent of renal cancer. Boys and girls are equally affected. The average age at which it is detected is 2 to 3 years. This neoplasm is significantly associated with birth defects such as aniridia and hemihypertrophy. Children with Wilms' tumor and aniridia often have deletion of a segment of a short arm of chromosome 11. Nephroblastoma originates from cells of the metanephrogenic blastema. Grossly the nephroblastoma is grayish white, soft and brain-like. It begins in the renal cortex and eventually replaces almost the entire kidney. Microscopically there are sheets of closely packed, atypical spindle cells within which there are embedded well-formed tubular or rosette-like structures. Glomeruloid structures are present. Smooth or striated muscle or cartilage may be present. In about 10 percent of cases, the neoplasm occurs bilaterally. Metastases are common in the lungs, liver, brain, and regional lymph nodes.

Papillary transitional cell carcinoma is by far the most common type of epithelial cancer occurring in the bladder. Cystoscopically a papillary mass is seen on the bladder wall. There is a significantly high incidence of bladder carcinoma in workers exposed to aniline dyes, benzidine, and α- and β-naphthylamine, in patients with schistosomiasis of the bladder, and among heavy cigarette smokers. Grossly, the neoplasm usually is a pink, delicately fronded, soft papillary mass growing from the bladder mucosa. The most highly malignant ones are firm and verrucous or flat and ulcerated. About half of these neoplasms arise in the trigone. Microscopically, the papillary folds have a thin fibrous core and are lined by several to many layers of transitional cells.

The lesions in uremia are quite variable and unpredictable. Most cases show only a few of the many changes associated with uremia. The brain may show marked edema. A fibrinous pericarditis is common, and fibrinous pleuritis occasionally occurs in severe renal insufficiency. In uremic pneumonitis, there are intra-alveolar hemorrhage and an accumulation of protein-rich fluid. Hyaline membranes line numerous alveolar walls. In the gastrointestinal tract there may be a stomatitis and necrotizing and ulcerative enterocolitis. Massive hemorrhage may result from the ulcerations. Patients who have been on long term dialysis often have multiple cysts in the kidneys. Hemorrhages (due to platelet dysfunction) and anemia (due to failure of erythropoietin production and to bone marrow depression and hemolysis caused by toxic metabolites) are commonly associated with chronic renal failure.

CHAPTER VII

REPRODUCTIVE PATHOLOGY

374.   A 20 year-old man began to have purulent urethral discharge. Gram-negative diplococci were found within neutrophils in a smear, and gonorrhea was diagnosed. Complications of gonorrhea in males include all of the following **EXCEPT**:

   (A)   acute epididymitis
   (B)   acute prostatitis
   (C)   phimosis
   (D)   septic arthritis
   (E)   urethral stricture

375.   A 30 year-old male prostitute developed severe constipation and passed only cigarette-sized fecal masses. The most likely cause is

   (A)   AIDS
   (B)   carcinoma of the rectum
   (C)   granuloma inguinale
   (D)   lymphopathia venereum
   (E)   syphilis

376.   A 60 year-old man developed urinary frequency and retained residual urine. Digital rectal examination revealed a nodular prostate which was neither hard nor fixed. His serum prostate specific antigen (PSA) level was 1.5 units. The likeliest diagnosis is

   (A)   acute prostatitis
   (B)   adenocarcinoma of prostate
   (C)   hyperplasia of prostate
   (D)   chronic prostatitis
   (E)   tuberculous prostatitis

377. On a routine examination a 65 year-old man was found to have a prostate specific antigen level of 52 units in his blood. Further studies revealed a prostatic adenocarcinoma. All of the following statements concerning prostatic cancer are correct **EXCEPT** that it

(A) is causally related to sexual promiscuity
(B) is not causally related to prostatic hyperplasia
(C) frequently metastasizes to bones
(D) may be associated with an elevated serum acid phosphatase
(E) often develops in the posterior lobe of the prostate

378. After puberty the most frequent complication of cryptorchidism is

(A) atrophy of the undescended testis
(B) development of a neoplasm in the undescended testis
(C) gynecomastia
(D) femoral hernia
(E) varicocele

379. Germinal neoplasms of the testis include all of the following **EXCEPT**:

(A) choriocarcinoma
(B) embryonal carcinoma
(C) Leydig cell tumor
(D) seminoma
(E) teratocarcinoma

380. All of the following are true concerning seminoma of the testis **EXCEPT** that it

(A) arises from a germ cell
(B) is highly malignant and metastasizes early
(C) is highly sensitive to radiation therapy
(D) is relatively more common in undescended than in scrotal testes
(E) is frequently infiltrated by lymphocytes

156

A 22 year-old medical student felt a painless, firm mass in his left testis. The testis was surgically removed. Low and high power photomicrographs of the tumor are shown in Figure 7.1.

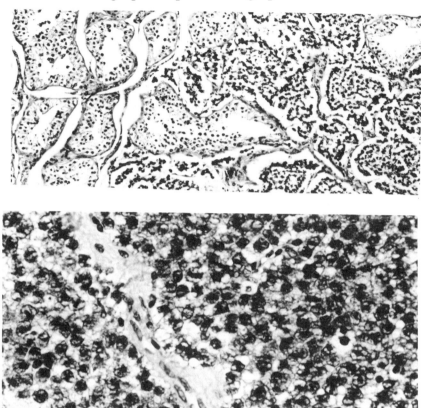

Figure 7.1

381. The likeliest diagnosis is

  (A)   choriocarcinoma
  (B)   embryonal carcinoma
  (C)   Leydig cell tumor
  (D)   seminoma
  (E)   teratocarcinoma

ANSWERS AND TUTORIAL ON ITEMS 374-381

The answers are: **374-C; 375-D; 376-C; 377-A; 378-A; 379-C; 380-B; 381-D**. <u>Neisseria gonorrhoeae</u> causes gonorrhea. The organism is spread by sexual contact. In males, there is a purulent discharge from the urethral orifice. Hematogenous complications include: septic arthritis, keratoderma blennorrhagica, in which there are vesicular lesions, which later show marked hyperkeratosis, on the feet, legs, trunk, arms, and face, and acute bacterial endocarditis, rarely. Genitourinary complications of gonorrhea in men are frequent in inadequately treated patients. They include urethral stricture, acute prostatitis, and acute epididymitis. All of these complications result from direct extension from the urethral infection. Phimosis is an inability to draw the prepuce back over the glans penis unrelated to gonorrhea.

The cause of lymphogranuloma (lymphopathia) venereum is Chlamydia trachomatis. Transmission is by sexual contact, especially in conditions of uncleanliness. The primary lesion is a small, indurated vesicular nodule on the prepuce. This usually ulcerates. The primary lesion is transient and disappears after a few days. Within 2 to 8 weeks inguinal lymph nodes enlarge to form buboes. In male homosexuals, anorectal infection may occur. Early there is a proctitis with a mucopurulent discharge, shallow ulcers of the mucosa, and the formation of polypoid masses on the mucosa. Rectal stricture follows the proctitis and is usually within 6 cm. of the anus. The rectal wall is thick, fibrous, and rigid, and the lumen is greatly narrowed.

Prostatic hyperplasia is the commonest cause of urinary obstruction in men over 50. The normal PSA rules out prostatic carcinoma in Item 376. However, in Item 377, the elevated PSA points to carcinoma, which is not related to sexual promiscuity.

Adenocarcinoma of the prostate gland seldom occurs in men under 50. The cause is unknown. Carcinoma is not causally related to prostatic hyperplasia. The prostate specific antigen is elevated. The serum level of acid phosphatase, which is formed largely by prostatic epithelial cells, is increased in cases with metastases. Serum alkaline phosphatase is also increased due to new bone formation. About 75 percent of prostatic carcinomas arise in the posterior lobe. Grossly, the lesion is grayish white with yellow spots; it is hard and is indistinctly demarcated from the surrounding tissue. Microscopically, there are small, fairly well differentiated glandular structures lined by atypical epithelium. The glands lie back to back with little or no intervening stroma. Metastases are frequent. Iliac and periaortic lymph nodes are involved in about 75 percent of the fatal cases; osseous metastases are present in up to 70 percent, the pelvic bones and sacrum almost always being involved in such cases. The bony metastases are osteoblastic.

Cryptorchidism is the failure of one or both testes to descend into the scrotal sac. The involved testis may have stopped in its downward descent anywhere along its path from the coelomic cavity to the inguinal canal. The cause is not always apparent. Cryptorchidism occurs in about 1 percent of males. Until puberty the undescended testis remains normal, but after puberty a gradually progressive atrophy with hyaline thickening of the tubular basement membranes, loss of germinal cells, and interstitial fibrosis occurs. Thus bilateral cryptorchidism in the adolescent or the young adult produces sterility. The undescended testis is roughly 15 times as likely to develop a neoplasm as is the normal scrotal testis.

Seminoma is the least malignant germinal neoplasm of the testes, and its pure form constitutes about 40 percent of such tumors. Grossly, the affected testis is partly or completely replaced by a firm, resilient, gray or tan mass with a glistening, bulging cut surface. Foci of necrosis are common. Microscopically, the seminoma consists of sheets of polyhedral cells which uniformly measure about 20μ in diameter. Fibrous trabeculae lobulate the neoplasm, and the fibrous stroma is typically infiltrated with lymphocytes. Metastases are most commonly to the periaortic and iliac lymph nodes, liver, and lungs. The 5-year survival rate is about 90 percent. Seminomas are highly sensitive to radiation.

Items 382-392

382. Complications of gonorrhea in females include all of the following **EXCEPT**:

    (A) acute salpingitis
    (B) Bartholin gland abscess
    (C) keratoconjunctivitis in newborn
    (D) septic arthritis
    (E) urethral caruncle

383. A 20 year-old woman had cramping lower abdominal pain which was exacerbated during her menstrual periods. Bilateral acute salpingitis was diagnosed. Complications of this condition include all of the following **EXCEPT**:

    (A) infertility
    (B) intestinal obstruction due to adhesions
    (C) pyosalpinx
    (D) rectal stricture
    (E) tubo-ovarian abscess

384. The commonest neoplasm of the female genital tract is

    (A) carcinoma of the cervix (in situ or invasive)
    (B) carcinoma of the endometrium
    (C) dermoid cyst of the ovary
    (D) leiomyoma of the uterus
    (E) serous cystadenoma of the ovary

385. Of the following, the pathologic change in a 20 year-old woman which has been significantly associated with intrauterine exposure to diethylstilbestrol is

    (A) adenocarcinoma of endometrium
    (B) clear cell adenocarcinoma of vagina
    (C) endometriosis
    (D) leiomyomata of uterus
    (E) serous cystadenoma of ovary

386. Of the following, the woman with the highest risk of developing cervical carcinoma is the one who

   (A)   had a mother who had cervical carcinoma
   (B)   had her menarche at 11 and menopause at 51
   (C)   has 6 children, the first being born when she was 16
   (D)   is a lesbian
   (E)   received estrogen therapy for menopausal problems

387. The usual cause of death in fatal cases of cervical carcinoma is

   (A)   hepatic failure due to liver metastases
   (B)   hypercalcemia due to bone metastases
   (C)   intestinal obstruction
   (D)   pulmonary embolism
   (E)   uremia due to urinary obstruction and infection

388. A 60 year-old woman developed vaginal bleeding. Uterine curettage revealed that she had endometrial adenocarcinoma. An increased incidence of carcinoma of the endometrium is associated with all of the following **EXCEPT**:

   (A)   diabetes mellitus
   (B)   menopausal and postmenopausal estrogen therapy
   (C)   hypertension
   (D)   multiparity
   (E)   obesity

389. All of the following are commonly found in benign cystic teratoma (dermoid cyst) of the ovary **EXCEPT**:

   (A)   chorionic villi
   (B)   hair
   (C)   sebaceous glands
   (D)   stratified squamous epithelium
   (E)   thyroid follicles

390. During an infertility work-up a 30 year-old woman was found to have enlarged ovaries with "chocolate cysts". The most likely diagnosis is

   (A)   corpora hemorrhagica
   (B)   endometriosis
   (C)   hemorrhage into serous cystadenomas
   (D)   dermoid cysts
   (E)   metastatic melanoma

160

391. A 25 year-old woman consulted her gynecologist because of infertility. The work-up revealed that she had the Stein-Leventhal syndrome. Features of this disorder include all of the following **EXCEPT**:

(A)   elevated androgen levels
(B)   increased incidence of ovarian cancer
(C)   menstrual irregularity
(D)   obesity
(E)   polycystic ovaries

392. An 8 year-old girl developed breasts and axillary and pubic hair. Estrogen levels were increased. Pelvic examination revealed a right ovarian mass. The most likely diagnosis is

(A)   benign cystic teratoma
(B)   Brenner tumor
(C)   choriocarcinoma
(D)   dysgerminoma
(E)   granulosa-theca cell tumor

ANSWERS AND TUTORIAL ON ITEMS 382-392

The answers are: **382-E; 383-D; 384-D; 385-B; 386-C; 387-E; 388-D; 389-A; 390-B; 391-B; 392-E**.

Gonorrheal complications in females may be by spread to vulval glands and internal genitalia or to joints hematogenously. During birth, gonococci may infect the newborn's eyes causing a keratoconjunctivitis.

Acute salpingitis does not lead to rectal stricture, which is a complication of lymphopathia venereum.

The uterine leiomyoma occurs in about a third of all women, being the most common internal neoplasm.

Cervical cancer is more common in women who begin sexual activity early in their teens and have multiple partners and pregnancies. Stage 4 carcinoma extends to surround the ureters and causes bilateral urinary obstruction and failure. Endometrial carcinoma on the other hand occurs in older women who have had no or few children.

In endometriosis externa, the ectopic glands respond to hormonal activity and bleed at menstrual periods, causing hemorrhagic cysts in the ovaries.

Dermoid cysts are made up mainly of tissues derived from ectoderm or endoderm. They contain no placental villi. Granulosa-theca cell tumors secrete estrogens and can produce isosexual precocious pseudopuberty in girls.

The initial stages of gonorrhea in the female usually consists of acute inflammation of the urethral meatus and of the mucous glands in the genital area (the periurethral (Skene's) glands and vulvovaginal (Bartholin's) glands), and marked edema and reddening of the mucosa, with pouting of the external os of the cervix. Infection of Bartholin's glands may go on to abscess formation (Bartholin abscess), or the infection may subside, to be followed by stricture of the ducts and, at a later date, cyst formation (Bartholin cyst).

Gonococcal keratoconjunctivitis usually occurs in children, although it may complicate gonorrhea in adults. It is most common in newborn infants (ophthalmia neonatorum), infection occurring during passage through the birth canal. In gonococcal keratoconjunctivitis, there is a severe acute purulent inflammation of the conjunctiva with ulceration of the cornea. This heals by fibrous scar formation, resulting in a corneal opacity which may produce blindness.

Salpingitis (inflammation of the uterine tube) is the most important genital complication of acute gonococcal infection in the female. Neisseria gonorrhoeae causes about half of cases of acute pelvic inflammatory disease, PID. Other causes are streptococci, Escherichia coli, anaerobic bacteria, and Chlamydia trachomatis. In salpingitis, at first the tubes are swollen and hyperemic, and the lateral ends leak a small amount of exudate into the peritoneal cavity, causing pelvic peritonitis. Later the fimbriae are agglutinated by fibrin deposits, the tubes become closed at both ends, and a purulent exudate accumulates in the lumen, giving "pus tubes" (pyosalpinx). If salpingitis develops at about the time of ovulation, the causative organism may infect the open lesion on the surface of the ovary, the fimbriae of the tube surrounding the follicle so that tube and ovary become involved together, causing salpingo-oöphoritis (tubo-ovarian abscess). With time the exudate slowly changes character until it becomes serous (hydrosalpinx). Often there are several acute exacerbations of the tubal infection, eventually followed by dense pelvic adhesions. The adhesions may cause periodic attacks of partial intestinal obstruction. Frequently they interfere with follicle development and ovulation, resulting in painful, irregular menstrual periods, and infertility. In those patients in whom ovulation continues, the tubal disease will often interfere with the migration of the fertilized ovum, resulting in ectopic pregnancy.

Vaginal adenosis, the presence of glandular epithelium in the submucosa of the upper vagina, has occurred in a large number of young women who were exposed to diethylstilbestrol in utero before the 18th week of pregnancy. Some of these women have developed clear cell adenocarcinoma of the vagina and cervix.

Despite early detection by means of Papanicolaou smears, carcinoma of the cervix is still an important cause of cancer deaths in the U.S. Cervical cancer is rare in nulliparas, occurring chiefly in women who have had many pregnancies, and especially in those having pregnancies early in life. The neoplasm is rare in virgins and in marital partners of males circumcised in infancy. Human papillomavirus may be related to the development of cervical carcinoma. Cigarette smoking is significantly associated with cervical carcinoma in situ. About 95 percent of cases are epidermoid carcinoma.

Cervical carcinoma usually begins at or near the squamocolumnar junction of the external orifice of the cervix. At first (stage 0) the neoplastic changes are confined to the surface epithelium (carcinoma in situ). After a long period of surface growth, apparently lasting 8 to 10 years, the malignant cells penetrate the basement membrane and infiltrate the submucosa (stage I). In stage II, the cells infiltrate between the muscle bundles of the cervix to reach the parametrium, and within the mucosa to involve the entire surface of the cervix and the upper portion of the vagina. In stage III, the ulcerating, fungating lesion extends downward to involve

162

the lower third of the vagina, and laterally in the parametrium to reach the pelvic walls. The final stage, stage IV, is reached when the neoplastic cells have extended locally to involve the bladder and rectum, have penetrated lymphatic channels to reach the pelvic lymph nodes, or have set up metastases in distant organs. Vesicovaginal or rectovaginal fistulae may develop during this phase. Especially important is the tendency to infiltrate the lymphatics surrounding the lower portion of the ureters, resulting in blockage of the urinary tract and hydronephrosis. Urinary tract infection and uremia are the usual terminal events in cervical cancer.

The most common malignant neoplasm of the body or fundus of the uterus is adenocarcinoma of the endometrium. The patient with endometrial carcinoma is generally first seen at about age 55 to 60, and her usual symptom is irregular vaginal bleeding. Obese women and women who have hypertension and/or diabetes mellitus are especially prone to endometrial cancer. The patients are often single or nulliparous, if married. Women given estrogens during the menopause or postmenopausal period have a significantly increased risk of developing endometrial carcinoma. Progestins are protective against these cancers when given along with estrogens. The use of combination oral contraceptives significantly reduces the risk of developing endometrial cancer.

Grossly, in endometrial carcinoma thickening of the endometrium develops, often bulging into the uterine cavity as a polyp, which is soft, friable, and vascular. Microscopically, the neoplasm is usually a well-differentiated adenocarcinoma with variably sized endometrial glands lined by atypical epithelium. Most endometrial carcinomas grow relatively slowly. In its late stages, the neoplastic cells will penetrate to the serosa and seed over the pelvic peritoneum to the pelvic and retroperitoneal lymph nodes, and to the submucosa of the urinary bladder, rectum, and ureters. Distant metastases are mainly to the lungs and liver.

The leiomyoma (fibroid) of the uterus arises from the smooth muscle cells of the myometrium. This neoplasm first appears during active sex life, grows during pregnancy, and regresses after menopause. Leiomyomas are often multiple. They may occur in any part of the uterus, but are most frequent in the body. Leiomyomas are white nodules, having a watered-silk appearance on cut section. They may compress their blood supply, causing infarction (red degeneration), especially during pregnancy. After the menopause or after infarction, they may undergo cystic or hyaline changes. The usual microscopic appearance is that of bundles of normal appearing smooth muscle fibers running in all directions.

Polycystic ovaries are present in the Stein-Leventhal syndrome: obesity, menstrual irregularity, variable masculinization, and infertility. The syndrome usually appears in the early twenties. Microscopically, there are numerous follicle cysts beneath a collagenized stroma. The cause of Stein-Leventhal syndrome is unclear. Elevated levels of androgens are secreted by the ovaries and adrenal cortex. Atypical hyperplasia or carcinoma of the endometrium occur in some cases, possibly due to peripheral conversion of androgens to estrogens.

Grossly, endometriosis externa is usually evident as multiple, reddish-brown or purple cystic nodules a few millimeters in diameter. These nodules are found on the surface of the ovaries, over the posterior surface of the uterus, or in the cul-de-sac. In the ovaries, the cysts often become somewhat larger, even several centimeters in diameter, and are filled with a thick, reddish-brown, pasty material ("chocolate cysts"). Microscopically, the cystic lesions are lined, at least in part, with recognizable endometrial tissue containing both glands and stroma. In endometriosis interna (adenomyosis), the misplaced endometrium is in the myometrium, the endometrial tissues being interlaced with smooth muscle fibers so as to form solid areas of thickening of the uterine wall adjoining the uterine cavity. These deep-lying nests of endometrium are composed of basal-type glands that do not respond to ovarian hormones. Therefore menstrual changes do not occur in them.

The dermoid cyst (benign cystic teratoma) arises from an ovum by parthenogenesis after the first meiotic division. It contains fatty material which is the secretion of the sebaceous glands in the skin lining of the wall of the cyst. Numerous hairs are present. The cyst wall usually shows a small mass bulging into the cavity. Near this mass the cyst often shows a thickening of the wall. Teeth, cartilage, and bone can frequently be identified in this tissue. Microscopically, a number of other well-differentiated but somewhat unorganized tissues can be made out, such as respiratory tract epithelium, thyroid tissue, gastric mucosa, salivary glands, dermal glands, neural tissue, and retina. The struma ovarii consists largely or entirely of thyroid tissue. In about 20 percent of the cases, dermoid cysts are bilateral.

The granuloma-theca cell tumor is a feminizing tumor due to elaboration of estrogen. It is usually unilateral, and is solid and yellow on cross section. Microscopically, it may show rosettes of small granular cells having ova-like structures (Call-Exner bodies), or it may have a cylindromatous pattern. The theca cells are lipid-containing cells resembling fibrous connective tissues. If the neoplasm appears in childhood, it may cause endometrial hyperplasia and bleeding, breast enlargement, growth of pubic and axillary hair, bone growth, and elevated estrogen levels. When this tumor appears during active sex life, no endocrine effects may be noted. If it develops after the menopause, it may cause endometrial hyperplasia or carcinoma and irregular uterine bleeding.

393. A breast lesion which usually appears during lactation is

    (A)   abscess
    (B)   fibrocystic mastopathy
    (C)   intraductal papilloma
    (D)   Paget's disease of the nipple
    (E)   sclerosing adenosis

394. A 30 year-old woman was in an automobile accident in which her right breast struck the steering wheel. Within a month a 3 cm. firm mass developed in the breast. The likeliest diagnosis is

    (A)   abscess
    (B)   carcinoma
    (C)   fat necrosis
    (D)   fibrous mastopathy
    (E)   plasma cell mastitis

395. A 45 year-old woman noted bleeding from her left nipple. A 2.5 cm. subareolar mass was felt. Nipple bleeding may occur in all of the following **EXCEPT**:

    (A)   intraductal papilloma
    (B)   intraductal carcinoma
    (C)   Paget's disease of the breast
    (D)   papillary adenocarcinoma
    (E)   medullary carcinoma

396. A 60 year-old woman had a firm, fixed 2 cm. mass in her right breast. This is most likely

    (A)   fibroadenoma
    (B)   fibrocystic mastopathy
    (C)   carcinoma
    (D)   periductal mastitis
    (E)   sclerosing adenosis

A 25 year-old woman felt a rubbery, movable 2 cm. mass in her right breast. It was removed surgically. A photomicrograph of the lesion is shown in Figure 7.2.

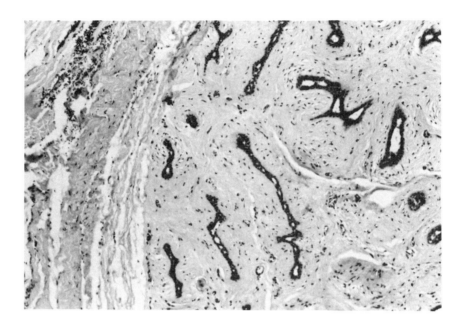

Figure 7.2

397.   This is most likely diagnosis is

   (A)   fibroadenoma
   (B)   fibrocystic mastopathy
   (C)   carcinoma
   (D)   periductal mastitis
   (E)   sclerosing adenosis

398.   A 65 year-old woman had a hard, fixed 2 cm. mass in her left breast. Clinically and on mammography it was diagnosed as a carcinoma. The most common type of breast carcinoma is

   (A)   infiltrating duct carcinoma with fibrosis
   (B)   intraductal carcinoma
   (C)   lobular carcinoma
   (D)   medullary carcinoma
   (E)   papillary carcinoma

399. All of the following appear to be risk factors in the development of breast carcinoma **EXCEPT**:

    (A)   early and frequent pregnancies
    (B)   exposure of the breast to X-radiation
    (C)   having a mother and/or sister with breast cancer
    (D)   high fat intake in the diet
    (E)   menopausal or postmenopausal estrogen therapy

ANSWERS AND TUTORIAL ON ITEMS 393-399

The answers are: **393-A; 394-C; 395-E; 396-C; 397-A; 398-A; 399-A**. Acute mastitis is practically limited to the period of lactation, especially during the first few weeks and in the primiparous. The causative agent (usually Staphylococcus aureus, less commonly Streptococci) invades the breast through fissures in the nipple, making its way via lymphatics or along ducts. Staphylococci tend to cause the development of one or more breast abscesses. With streptococcal mastitis there is a diffuse acute inflammation of the breast.

Fat necrosis is a quiet degeneration of the adipose tissue of the breast, which is due to trauma, including surgical biopsy and X-radiotherapy for breast cancer. Grossly, the lesion is well defined, firm solid, chalky, and lard-like early. Microscopically, early there are opaque fat cells, and the adipose tissue is infiltrated by neutrophils, plasmacytes, lymphocytes, and macrophages. Epithelioid, foam, and giant cells may be found. Later there is necrosis, with cholesterol crystals, fibrosis, and calcification.

Fibroadenoma is a very common, slowly growing, estrogen-induced, fibroepithelial neoplasm, usually occurring in women between 25 and 35 years of age. Growth is rapid during pregnancy and lactation and usually ceases at the menopause. The skin over the fibroadenoma is unchanged, and it is movable under the skin. Grossly, the tumor feels rubbery and is smooth or lobulated, sharply outlined, encapsulated, and 0.5 to 3.5 cm. in diameter. The color is pearly-gray or pink. The cut surface is delicately fissured by ducts and feels moist or sticky. Old tumors may show hyalinization or calcification.

Nipple bleeding occurs in neoplasms which occur in subareolar ducts, especially papillary tumors which are friable. Paget's disease is characterized by an intraductal carcinoma from which cells migrate up a duct to involve the nipple mucosa.

Carcinoma of the breast occurs in about one in 9 women in the United States. Most breast carcinomas are discovered shortly before, during, or just after the menopause. In general, the older the patient, the more likely a single lump in the breast is carcinoma. While the cause of breast carcinoma is not completely known, three factors appear to play an important role: heredity, hormones, and diet. Hereditary factors appear more prominently in relation to breast carcinoma than in most types of cancer. The risk of developing breast carcinoma is two to three times higher in women whose mothers or sisters have had this disease than would be expected. Prolonged estrogen stimulation acts as a promoter for the development of breast carcinoma. In women with an early menarche and late menopause (and thus an extended exposure of cyclic stimulation of breast epithelium by estrogens), the incidence of mammary cancer is greater than in those with a shorter span of ovarian activity. Breast carcinoma is significantly more common among unmarried than married women and among nulliparous than parous women. A late first pregnancy may increase the risk. A slightly increased risk of breast cancer has been found in women with prolonged estrogen use (> 20 years) as compared to controls. The use of oral contraceptives does not appear to increase the incidence of breast cancer. Nutritional factors, especially a high total fat intake, have been implicated in the causation of mammary cancer. Ionizing radiation appears to be a cause of breast carcinoma. Rarely it has occurred in women exposed to repeated fluoroscopic examinations of the chest. The incidence of mammary carcinoma in women exposed to over 90 rads in the atomic bombing in Japan has been about four times the expected rate.

Infiltrating duct carcinoma with fibrosis (scirrhous carcinoma) is the most common type of carcinoma in the breast, constituting about 75 percent of all mammary carcinomas. Grossly, the scirrhous carcinoma averages 2 cm. in diameter and is very hard, fixed to the surrounding breast tissue, and tan with yellow streaks. It cuts with the grittiness of unripe fruit. The cut surface is concave and retracts below the level of the cut. Microscopically, there is marked fibrosis with minute, angular, cleft-like spaces containing closely packed atypical epithelial cells in thin columns or threads.

Items 400-410

400.   The commonest site of ectopic pregnancy is the

(A)   cervix uteri
(B)   ovary
(C)   pelvic peritoneum
(D)   uterine tube
(E)   vagina

401.   Conditions which predispose to the development of tubal pregnancy include all of the following **EXCEPT**:

(A)   chronic salpingitis
(B)   endometriosis
(C)   leiomyomata of uterus
(D)   peritubal adhesions following pelvic peritonitis
(E)   successful tubal ligation

168

402. A 20 year-old woman who was 3 months pregnant aborted a mass which resembled a bunch of grapes. It was identified as a complete hydatidiform mole. All of the following are true statements about this disorder **EXCEPT**:

(A) it is caused by fertilization of an ovum without chromosomes
(B) it has a diploid 46XX pattern
(C) almost all chorionic villi are cystic
(D) there is trophoblastic proliferation
(E) there is little tendency to develop choriocarcinoma

403. All of the following statements concerning partial hydatidiform mole are true **EXCEPT**:

(A) the cause is the fertilization of an ovum by two sperms
(B) the karyotype is triploid 69XXY
(C) fetal parts may be present
(D) only some chorionic villi are cystic
(E) human chorionic gonadotropin levels are not elevated

404. All of the following statements concerning choriocarcinoma are true **EXCEPT**:

(A) about half the cases in women arise in a hydatidiform mole
(B) the neoplastic cells produce high titers of chorionic gonadotropin
(C) both cyto- and syncytiotrophoblastic cells are present microscopically
(D) hematogenous metastases to the lungs are common
(E) the prognosis is better in testicular than placental choriocarcinoma

405. A woman in her third trimester of pregnancy became comatose and went into premature labor. Toxemia of pregnancy was diagnosed. All of the following are characteristic of eclampsia **EXCEPT**:

(A) edema due to protein loss in the urine
(B) hypertension
(C) maternal diabetes is a predisposing factor
(D) premature separation of the placenta
(E) subcapsular and parenchymal hemorrhages in the liver

406. Predisposing factors in the development of chorioamnionitis include all of the following **EXCEPT**:

   (A) cervical incompetence
   (B) cervical or vaginal instrumentation late in pregnancy
   (C) coitus late in pregnancy
   (D) maternal bacteremia
   (E) prolonged rupture of fetal membranes

407. Of the following the one most likely to be associated with fetal exsanguination is

   (A) abruptio placentae (premature placental separation)
   (B) formation of a tight knot in the umbilical cord
   (C) placenta praevia
   (D) single umbilical artery
   (E) velamentous insertion of the umbilical cord

408. A full term fetus died during labor. Findings at autopsy that the death was due to fetal anoxia include all of the following **EXCEPT**:

   (A) amniotic fluid debris in lungs
   (B) meconium staining of the fetal membranes
   (C) opacification of the fetal membranes
   (D) large infarct of the placenta
   (E) subepicardial and subpleural petechiae

409. All of the following are causes of fetal anoxia **EXCEPT**:

   (A) abruptio placentae
   (B) formation of a tight knot in the umbilical cord
   (C) placenta praevia
   (D) single umbilical artery
   (E) velamentous insertion of the umbilical cord with rupture of a large velamentous blood vessel

410. After breathing apparently normally for 24 hours, an infant developed respiratory distress due to hyaline membrane disease. Predisposing factors to the development of this condition include all of the following **EXCEPT**:

   (A) cesarean section
   (B) maternal diabetes
   (C) prematurity
   (D) respiratory viral infection
   (E) second born of twins

170

ANSWERS AND TUTORIAL ON ITEMS 400-410

The answers are: **400-D; 401-E; 402-E; 403-E; 404-E; 405-C; 406-D; 407-E; 408-C; 409-D; 410-D**.

Most ectopic pregnancies occur in a uterine tube. Any pathologic change which causes narrowing or blockage of the tubal lumen predisposes to tubal pregnancy. The narrowing may be intrinsic due to inflammation or extrinsic due to formation of adhesions around the tube. Tubal ligation is designed to prevent fertilization of ovum by sperm and thus any pregnancy.

Hydatidiform mole may be complete or partial. It is characterized by cystic chorionic villi. Choriocarcinoma may develop in a mole, especially the complete type. About 50 percent of gestational choriocarcinomas arise in moles. Many of these have been treated successfully with chemotherapy.

Eclampsia is a severe toxemia of pregnancy of uncertain cause. It is not related to maternal diabetes mellitus.

Chorioamnionitis is due to bacteria from the vagina, so any kind of instrumentation late in pregnancy predisposes to it. Chorioamnionitis is not related to maternal bacteremia.

Fetal exsanguination can result from rupture of a placental blood vessel when these are exposed by velamentous insertion into the fetal membranes instead of directly into the placental mass.

Fetal anoxia results from such exsanguination, separation of a significant portion of the placenta prematurely, or by compression of the umbilical cord.

Hyaline membrane disease occurs mainly in prematures because of immaturity of the lungs and absence of surfactant in the alveoli. Other clinical situations have been observed to predispose to its development, sometimes without obvious cause, in full term infants.

Tubal pregnancy is the most common form of ectopic pregnancy. It occurs about once in 200 pregnancies. The burrowing trophoblast usually erodes and ruptures the tube early in pregnancy. Sometimes tubal abortion occurs, the fetus being extruded from the lateral end of the tube into the abdominal cavity. Interstitial pregnancy is implantation in a cornu of the uterus in the interstitial portion of the uterine tube. "Abdominal" pregnancy (peritoneal pregnancy) may result either from direct implantation of the fertilized ovum upon the peritoneum or from extrusion of the fetus of a tubal pregnancy into the abdominal cavity. Ovarian pregnancy is extremely rare and presumably results from fertilization of the ovum at the time of ovulation.

A hydatidiform mole occurs once in about 2000 pregnancies. Its incidence is higher among women at the two extremes of maternal age than in other women. The serum and urinary chorionic gonadotropin levels are usually abnormally high. In complete mole, the cause is fertilization of an ovum which has lost its chromosomes. Almost all have a 46XX diploid pattern from the sperm by androgenesis. There are no fetal parts. Almost every chorionic villus is cystic and avascular. There is diffuse trophoblastic proliferation. About 2 percent develop choriocarcinoma. Partial mole is due to fertilization of an ovum by 2 sperms. It has a triploid 69XXY chromosomal pattern. Only some villi are cystic, and there is slight trophoblastic proliferation. Fetal parts may be present. Choriocarcinoma rarely develops from a partial mole. The first manifestation of the presence of a mole is often the excessively rapid enlargement of the uterus due to growth of the placental mass. This is usually followed, at about the third to fifth month of pregnancy, by uterine bleeding or abortion. Placental tissue passed at this time shows that the villi are cystic and grape-like. Microscopically, the mole shows cystic avascular villi together with irregular clumps of large syncytial and cytotrophoblastic cells.

Gestational choriocarcinoma is a rare neoplasm. In about half the cases, it arises in women with a hydatid mole. The remainder of the cases are about equally divided between abortions and full-term pregnancy. A few develop as a teratoma unrelated to a pregnancy. Grossly, the uterus containing a choriocarcinoma shows shaggy, fleshy hemorrhagic masses filling the uterine cavity and extending into the myometrium. Microscopically, the neoplasm is composed of clusters of large, bizarre, often multinucleated giant trophoblastic cells, extending into the myometrium and often filling the vascular sinuses. Necrosis and hemorrhage are seen, both in the tumor masses and in the myometrium. Very rarely both the primary neoplasm and the metastases have disappeared spontaneously. Numerous cures have been achieved by methotrexate and actinomycin D in choriocarcinomas related to a mole or pregnancy. Typically the tumor spreads locally to the vagina and parametrium, invades the veins, and metastasizes to the lungs, liver, and brain. Usually the neoplastic cells produce chorionic gonadotropin in both the primary growth and the metastases, sometimes with extremely high titers.

Toxemia of pregnancy is usually manifest by proteinuria, hypertension, visual impairment, and edema. In the most seriously affected patients, there may also be convulsions and coma. These characterize the disease known as eclampsia. Cases without convulsions and coma are referred to as preeclampsia. Premature labor is an important feature of the toxemias, due to the increased uterine contractility resulting from secretion of pituitary oxytocin. The increase in tonus and in contraction of the uterus causes a reduction of the maternal blood flow in the placenta and a tendency to separation of the placenta. These two factors, both of which would promote fetal anoxia, may account for the high fetal mortality in toxemia of pregnancy. The immediate cause of toxemia remains unknown.

In eclampsia the liver is enlarged and soft and has hemorrhages in the capsule and parenchyma. Microscopically, there are scattered areas of necrosis, which may be peripheral. The kidneys are swollen and may show petechiae. Microscopic changes are noted in the glomeruli (swelling of capillary basement membranes, capillary thrombosis) and in the tubules (epithelial swelling and degeneration). In extreme cases, bilateral renal cortical necrosis develops. Foci of placental infarction may be found. Microscopically, capillary thrombi and knots of syncytial trophoblasts are present in chorionic villi.

Chorioamnionitis is an infection of the fetal membranes. Predisposing factors include prolonged rupture of the membranes, prolonged labor, vaginal and/or cervical instrumentation, and placenta praevia. It is almost always an ascending infection from the lower genital tract. The common causes are gram-negative bacilli and streptococci. In chorioamnionitis, the membranes are thickened, dull and infiltrated with neutrophils. The amniotic fluid is cloudy and contains many neutrophils. A fetal pneumonitis may develop due to inhalation of infected amniotic fluid. Extension of the infection to the umbilical cord causes acute funicitis. Villous placentitis is infection of the chorionic villi due to hematogenous seeding by viruses, Treponema pallidum, Mycobacterium tuberculosis, or other bacteria from the maternal circulation. Fetal infection may result by extension from the placenta.

The umbilical cord is normally inserted somewhere near the center of the fetal surface of the placenta, but sometimes the cord is attached eccentrically or even at the very edge of the

172

placental mass (marginal attachment, battledore placenta). Rarely the placental vessels converge to form the cord in the membranes entirely outside the placental mass. This velamentous origin of the cord carries some danger for the fetus. If the rupture of the amniotic sac occurs through the region of these vessels, as in vasa praevia, it may cause fetal death from exsanguination.

Interference with fetal oxygenation is the most common cause of intrauterine death and of death during labor. Anoxia may be due to abnormalities of the placenta, such as premature separation or placenta praevia; to abnormalities of the umbilical cord, such as prolapse, knots, or entanglement; or to maternal anoxia, as from excessive sedation. Most of the abnormalities of the umbilical cord are mechanical and result in interference with blood flow in the cord. The cord may prolapse ahead of the fetus, in which case it may be compressed between the presenting part and the cervix. The cord may be twisted about the neck of the fetus as a result of intrauterine activity. Occasionally an overhand knot is formed in the cord. These complications, more common with twins than with single pregnancies, may cause fetal anoxia and death.

Hyaline membrane disease is a common cause of death in newborn infants, especially prematures, the second born of twins, those with fetal hypoxia, those delivered by cesarean section, and those born of diabetic mothers. The newborn infant respires normally for 8 to 24 hours. After that time respirations become labored and accelerated, and dyspnea and cyanosis appear. Death usually occurs within 24 to 48 hours.

In the premature infant the biochemical pathways for the formation of surfactant, dipalmitoyl phosphatidylcholine, by type 2 pneumocytes along the alveolar septa are not fully developed. Deficiency of surfactant, which has a detergent-like effect along alveolar membranes, results in hyaline membrane formation. Immaturity of the fibrinolytic enzyme system in the premature is an important predisposing factor for the development of fibrin membranes. Grossly, the lungs are reddish purple and extensively atelectatic. Microscopically, eosinophilic fibrin membranes line respiratory bronchioles and alveolar ducts. Most alveoli and many alveolar ducts are collapsed.

Items 411-416

411. Features of Turner's syndrome include all of the following **EXCEPT**:

   (A)   increased incidence of leukemia
   (B)   infantile genitalia
   (C)   ovarian agenesis (streak ovaries)
   (D)   short stature
   (E)   45,X karyotype

412. All of the following are characteristic of Klinefelter's syndrome **EXCEPT**:

(A) gynecomastia
(B) increased incidence of testicular neoplasm
(C) low normal intelligence
(D) small testes
(E) XXY sex chromosome pattern

413. All of the following are features of Down's syndrome **EXCEPT**:

(A) most cases have trisomy 21
(B) most patients develop Alzheimer's disease by 35 years
(C) there is frequently a webbed neck
(D) there is an increased incidence of acute leukemia
(E) there is an increased incidence of congenital heart defects

414. After an uneventful first pregnancy, a 25 year-old woman gave birth to a full term infant with anemia and jaundice. Erythroblastosis fetalis was diagnosed and exchange transfusion was performed with success. All of the following are true concerning erythroblastosis fetalis **EXCEPT**:

(A) the mother is Rh-negative and the fetus is Rh-positive
(B) the mother must be sensitized to Rh antigen
(C) the D antigen is the most important
(D) Rhogam (anti-D Ig) prevents sensitization when injected into the mother
(E) incompatibility in ABO groups never causes fetal erythroblastosis

415. All of the following statements about phenylketonuria are true **EXCEPT**:

(A) the disease is due to a deficiency of phenylalanine hydroxylase
(B) phenylalanine accumulates in the blood and cerebrospinal fluid
(C) mental deficiency is common
(D) melanin-like pigment is deposited in tissues
(E) patients with PKU may not use foods or drinks containing aspartame

416. The grandmother noticed that her 6 month old grandson tasted salty when kissed. The pediatrician diagnosed cystic fibrosis. All of the following are true statements about this disorder **EXCEPT**:

(A) it is transmitted as an autosomal recessive
(B) Caucasian children are most often affected
(C) there is widespread involvement of exocrine glands
(D) in infancy and childhood, pancreatic involvement dominates
(E) death is usually due to the development of juvenile diabetes mellitus

ANSWERS AND TUTORIAL ON ITEMS 411-416

The answers are: **411-A; 412-B; 413-C; 414-E; 415-D; 416-E**. In classic Turner's syndrome (ovarian dysgenesis), there are only 45 chromosomes, 1 sex chromosome being absent (XO). This syndrome includes bilateral ovarian agenesis (streak ovaries), infantile genitalia, short stature, short webbed neck, high arched palate, cardiovascular and renal defects (such as coarctation of the aorta and horseshoe kidney), and cubitus valgus (an outward deviation of the extended forearm). In Klinefelter's syndrome (testicular dysgenesis), there are 47 chromosomes due to the presence of an additional X sex chromosome (XXY). The features include atrophy of the testicular tubules with persistence of the interstitial cells and gynecomastia. Intelligence is in the low normal range.

In Down's syndrome there is typically trisomy on autosome 21. Down's syndrome occurs in sporadic, familial, and mosaic forms. Sporadic trisomy 21 makes up about 85 percent of the cases. It is most common in the offspring of women over 35 years of age. Trisomy 21 is due to nondisjunction during gametogenesis, usually oögenesis. The affected child has 47 chromosomes in the body cells. Familial mongolism is rare (about 2 percent of cases) and is more common in the offspring of young mothers. Patients with familial Down's syndrome have 46 chromosomes with reciprocal translocation of a small autosome, usually from 21, on chromosome 15. In Down's syndrome, the infant has a small brain with defective gyri and a reduced number of neurons; slanting eyes; white flecks in the irides (Brushfield spots); fat cheeks and back of the neck; a protruding tongue; short thumbs; square palms with a simian line; markedly hypotonic musculature; a wide gap between the first and second toes; sterility in males; and cardiac defects, especially interventricular septal defect and persistent atrioventricular ostium. Acute or subacute leukemia occurs commonly.

Erythroblastosis fetalis is a hemolytic disease. The fetal red blood cells are destroyed by a maternal agglutinin interacting in the fetus with a fetal agglutinogen which has been inherited from the father. The usual agglutinogen in erythroblastosis is the Rh factor, especially the D antigen. Rarely a fetal-maternal incompatibility in ABO blood groups may cause fetal erythroblastosis, but this form is seldom fatal. The mother can develop antibodies against the fetal Rh agglutinogen by fetal red cells leaking into the maternal circulation, thus sensitizing her by causing the formation of anti-Rh antibodies in her blood plasma. These anti-Rh antibodies diffuse through the placental barrier and enter the fetal circulation. There they coat the fetus' Rh-positive red cells, causing their intravascular hemolysis. Usually it takes one or two pregnancies with an Rh-positive fetus or one transfusion of Rh-positive blood to sensitize the mother. Hence, erythroblastosis usually appears in the second or later pregnancies, rarely in the first.

The blood picture is one of hemolytic anemia. There are large numbers of nucleated red cells both in blood smears and in tissue sections. The placenta, liver, and spleen are large. Enlargement of the placenta is due to edema, whereas extramedullary erythropoiesis is the chief cause for the enlargement of the liver and spleen. The kidneys are large and pale, and the tubules show epithelial degeneration and heme casts. The brain in infants living some hours shows marked icteric tinting of the basal ganglia (kernicterus) due to deposition of unconjugated bilirubin. In the placenta, the chorionic villi are edematous. Lipid-laden macrophages (Hofbauer cells) are found in the loose stroma of the villi. Rhogam (anti-D immunoglobulin) prevents Rh sensitization when it is injected into the mother postnatally.

Phenylketonuria (PKU) occurs about once in 10,000 births and in 1 percent of mental defectives. It is transmitted by a rare recessive gene. There is a block in the conversion of phenylalanine to tyrosine due to a deficiency of phenylalanine hydroxylase. Phenylalanine accumulates in the blood and cerebrospinal fluid. The excess is converted to phenylpyruvic acid. The phenylalanine in excess, or one of its products, damages neurons, producing mental deficiency and convulsions. Children with phenylketonuria are often blue-eyed blondes, the light skin and eye pigmentation being due to decreased melanin pigmentation. Aspartame contains phenylalanine and may not be used by phenylketonurics.

Cystic fibrosis (mucoviscidosis) is transmitted as an autosomal recessive. The defective gene is on the long arm of chromosome 7. About 95 percent of cases occur in Caucasians. The basic defect in cystic fibrosis is due to a mutation in the gene encoding for the cystic fibrosis transmembrane conductance regulator (CFTR), causing a defect in the transport of chloride ions across epithelium. The tracheobronchial mucous glands, pancreatic ducts, biliary canaliculi, salivary gland secretory epithelium, and sweat glands may be involved. In about 10 percent of the cases there are signs of intestinal obstruction at birth, due to meconium ileus. In most cases the disease is recognized some months or years after birth, either because of obvious nutritional deficiency or because of recurring respiratory infections of unusual severity and persistence. The sodium and chloride content of sweat is two to three times the normal level. Children with this disease often taste salty when kissed, and salt may precipitate on their foreheads after exertion. In cases surviving infancy, the pulmonary changes overshadow those of the pancreas clinically. Rarely do victims of this disease survive beyond young adulthood.

In fibrocystic disease, the pancreas is variable in size because of cysts which are often present. The parenchyma is atrophic and fibrous. Microscopically the acinar tissue is almost completely absent, but islets of Langerhans usually remain. In the pancreas, atrophy of acinar cells is apparently secondary to the inspissation within ducts of mucus secreted by goblet cells. In the liver there is cholangiolar proliferation behind inspissated mucus in intrahepatic biliary ducts. In children with severe degrees of pancreatic insufficiency, the feces become so bulky, inspissated, and putty-like as to cause intestinal obstruction mechanically or by intussusception. Bronchiectasis results from bronchial obstruction by highly viscous mucus and superimposed infection.

CHAPTER VIII

ENDOCRINE PATHOLOGY

Items 417-425

417. By the age of 16, a young man had grown to a height of 7½ feet. Skull films showed an enlargement of the sella turcica. Of the following, the most likely causative lesion is

    (A) acidophil adenoma of pituitary
    (B) basophil adenoma of pituitary
    (C) craniopharyngioma
    (D) pinealoma
    (E) pituitary adenocarcinoma

418. A 30 year-old man developed bilateral homonymous hemianopsia. He also had moderate enlargement of his lower jaw and hands. Of the following the likeliest cause is

    (A) adamantinoma
    (B) basophil adenoma of pituitary
    (C) chromophobe adenoma of pituitary
    (D) craniopharyngioma
    (E) glioma of optic chiasm

419. During labor a 25 year-old gravida 3 para 2 had a premature placental separation and lost 500 ml. of blood. Postpartum she developed panhypopituitarism. The cause of the hypopituitarism in Sheehan's syndrome is

    (A) chromophobe adenoma of pituitary
    (B) craniopharyngioma
    (C) hemorrhage into sella turcica
    (D) idiopathic atrophy of pituitary
    (E) infarction of pituitary

420. Causes of Cushing's syndrome include all of the following **EXCEPT**:

   (A)   adrenal cortical adenoma
   (B)   basophil adenoma of pituitary
   (C)   chromophobe adenoma of pituitary
   (D)   long-term adrenal corticosteroid therapy
   (E)   papillary carcinoma of thyroid

421. The most characteristic alteration in the anterior pituitary in Cushing's syndrome associated with a functional adrenal neoplasm is

   (A)   basophil adenoma
   (B)   chromophobe adenoma
   (C)   Crooke's hyaline degeneration of basophils
   (D)   infarction
   (E)   metastatic bronchogenic small cell carcinoma

422. The abnormal findings in Cushing's syndrome include all of the following **EXCEPT**:

   (A)   diabetes mellitus
   (B)   hypersexuality
   (C)   obesity, especially of face and trunk
   (D)   osteoporosis
   (E)   purplish striae in abdominal skin

423. The abnormal findings in Conn's syndrome include all of the following **EXCEPT**:

   (A)   adrenal cortical adenoma
   (B)   diabetes mellitus
   (C)   hyperaldosteronism
   (D)   hypertension
   (E)   hypokalemia

424. The finding of increased urinary catecholamines is characteristic of

   (A)   Addison's disease
   (B)   Cushing's syndrome
   (C)   medullary carcinoma of thyroid
   (D)   pheochromocytoma
   (E)   primary hyperaldosteronism

425. A 40 year-old Caucasian male became weak and easily fatigued. His skin and gingiva were tan, and his blood pressure was 110/60. Addison's disease was diagnosed. In chronic adrenal cortical insufficiency, the commonest adrenal lesion is

(A)   amyloidosis
(B)   histoplasmosis
(C)   idiopathic atrophy
(D)   metastatic carcinoma
(E)   tuberculosis

ANSWERS AND TUTORIAL ON ITEMS 417-425

The answers are: **417-A; 418-C; 419-E; 420-E; 421-C; 422-B; 423-B; 424-D; 425-C**.

Gigantism is due to excessive secretion of growth hormone by a neoplasm of the adenohypophysis before epiphyses are closed. This hormone is normally produced by acidophil cells, but is also secreted by some chromophobe adenomas. In adults, excessive growth hormone causes acromegaly with enlarged bones and viscera. Pituitary adenomas are histologically benign but may grow out of the sella turcica to compress the optic chiasm and produce bilateral homonymous hemianopsia.

Cushing's syndrome may be caused by ACTH-producing neoplasms of the pituitary or certain malignant tumors such as small cell bronchogenic carcinoma or by autonomous over-production of corticosteroids by an adrenal neoplasm or hyperplasia. It is also an iatrogenic disorder due to long term adrenocorticosteroid therapy. Crooke's hyaline change in basophils is a retrogressive change due to high levels of corticosteroids from an adrenal neoplasm or hyperplasia.

In Cushing's syndrome there is an over-production of the adrenal glucocorticoids. The syndrome is more common in females than in males. The usual manifestations are: (1) obesity, chiefly of the trunk and face; (2) skin disorders such as acne and purplish striae of the thighs and abdomen; (3) diminished sexual function (amenorrhea in females; impotence in males); (4) hypertension; (5) hirsutism in females; (6) diabetes mellitus, or more often a diabetic type of glucose tolerance curve; and (7) osteoporosis.

Primary hyperaldosteronism (Conn's syndrome) consists of hypertension, polyuria, hypokalemia, and severe muscle weakness, simulating paralysis. In most instances, it is associated with an adrenal cortical adenoma, occasionally with an adrenal carcinoma or adrenal hyperplasia. The adenomas consist almost entirely of zona glomerulosa cells or of a mixture of glomerulosa and fasciculata-type cells.

Increased production of the two hormones - epinephrine and mainly norepinephrine - of the adrenal medulla is usually due to tumor of the chromaffin cells (pheochromocytoma), but may be due to tumor of the related chromaffin bodies of the sympathetic nervous system. The characteristic manifestations are a result of paroxysmal hypertension. Increased levels of catecholamines appear in the urine.

Hyperfunction of the acidophil cells is usually a result of an eosinophilic adenoma. The hyperfunction is usually manifest by increased bone growth. When the condition arises before epiphyseal closure has occurred, it results in abnormal tallness or gigantism. When the hyperfunction has its onset after age 20, there is little opportunity for increase in height since the epiphyses of the long bones are already closed. Instead the bone growth is manifest by a general increase in bone mass, the condition being known as acromegaly. This is especially evident in the lower jaw (prognathism). The fingers broaden, and the hands become spade-like. The viscera are also enlarged. Some patients develop diabetes mellitus due to insulin resistance.

Simmond's disease (hypophyseal cachexia) is due to extreme hypofunction of the adenohypophysis. It is usually a result of a destructive process, either vascular or neoplastic. Vascular causes include infarction of the pituitary gland, usually due to prolonged circulatory failure following severe intrapartum or postpartum hemorrhage (Sheehan's syndrome). Neoplasms causing Simmond's disease may be primary, either in the pituitary gland or in adjacent structures or they may be metastatic, as from breast cancer. Chromophobe adenoma is the commonest cause. Congenital hypopituitarism occurs in boys twice as frequently as in girls. The child develops into a well-proportioned but short person (Lorain-Levi type). Hypopituitarism in children is usually due to a craniopharyngioma, a squamous neoplasm which destroys the pituitary by compression.

Pituitary adenomas vary in size from microscopic to 10 cm. in diameter. These may greatly enlarge the sella turcica and may compress nearby brain structures. After a certain size is reached, the neoplasm breaks through the diaphragma sella. Many structures may be compressed by the growing neoplasm, particularly the optic chiasm, nerves, and tracts, and the non-neoplastic cells of the gland. In most instances, pituitary neoplasms are encapsulated and are benign. Over half of these neoplasms are chromophobe adenomas, and most of the remainder are eosinophilic adenomas or mixed cellular types. Basophilic adenomas are uncommon.

Pheochromocytomas of the adrenal medulla are variable in size, ranging from 1 gm. to over 1 kg. Most are encapsulated, and on section they are pink and soft. Microscopically, they are composed of nests of polyhedral cells, usually constant in size and morphology. A fine network of fibers usually separates the cell nests. About 1 percent are malignant, and in about 10 percent of cases pheochromocytomas are bilateral.

Chronic adrenal cortical insufficiency (Addison's disease) occurs chiefly in middle life. In crisis, circulatory collapse may be profound. More than 90 percent of adrenal cortical cells must be lost before hypofunction becomes manifest. Tuberculosis of the adrenal glands is a common cause of Addison's disease. In such cases, both glands are almost totally destroyed. In recent years, idiopathic cortical atrophy of the glands has become the most important cause. It may be due to an autoimmune reaction. Anti-adrenal antibodies are found in the sera of over half the cases. The atrophic glands are reduced to as little as 2.5 gm. combined weight (normal 8 gm.). Occasionally Addison's disease is a result of histoplasmosis, bilateral adrenal metastases, especially from bronchogenic carcinoma, or of amyloid disease of the adrenal glands.

A 30 year-old woman became hyperactive and irritable. There was a mass in her neck, and her eyes protruded. A subtotal thyroidectomy was performed. A photograph of the thyroid is shown in Figure 8.1.

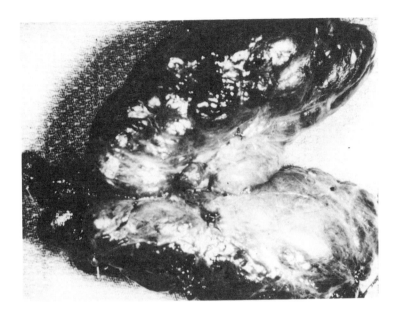

Figure 8.1

426.   The likeliest diagnosis is

    (A)   diffuse primary hyperplasia
    (B)   follicular carcinoma
    (C)   lymphocytic thyroiditis
    (D)   medullary carcinoma
    (E)   nodular goiter

427.   A 30 year-old multigravida became sluggish and developed myxedema. The causes of hypothyroidism include all of the following **EXCEPT**:

    (A)   autoantibodies to TSH receptors on follicular cells
    (B)   iodine deficiency in diet
    (C)   goitrogenic drugs
    (D)   lymphocytic thyroiditis
    (E)   thyroid carcinoma

428. All of the following are true statements about papillary carcinoma of the thyroid gland **EXCEPT**:

(A)   it is the commonest type of thyroid cancer
(B)   calcified psammoma bodies are found in papillae
(C)   it can be caused by X-rays
(D)   the nuclei of malignant cells have a pale "ground glass" appearance
(E)   it is highly malignant and metastasizes early

429. All of the following are true statements concerning medullary carcinoma of the thyroid gland **EXCEPT**:

(A)   it arises from parafollicular C cells
(B)   it contains stromal deposits of amyloid
(C)   it may elaborate excessive amounts of calcitonin
(D)   it may produce Cushing's syndrome by elaborating ACTH
(E)   it often arises in glands which are the site of lymphocytic thyroiditis

430. The commonest cause of secondary hyperparathyroidism is

(A)   calcitonin producing medullary thyroid carcinoma
(B)   chronic renal insufficiency
(C)   low dietary calcium intake
(D)   metastatic calcification
(E)   vitamin D deficiency

431. Systemic effects of hyperparathyroidism include all of the following **EXCEPT**:

(A)   demineralization of bones
(B)   metastatic calcification
(C)   nephrolithiasis
(D)   peptic ulcer
(E)   tetany

A 50 year-old woman was found to have a diffusely enlarged thyroid gland. Laboratory findings revealed a mild hypothyroidism. A surgical procedure was performed. A photomicrograph of the surgical specimen is shown in Figure 8.2.

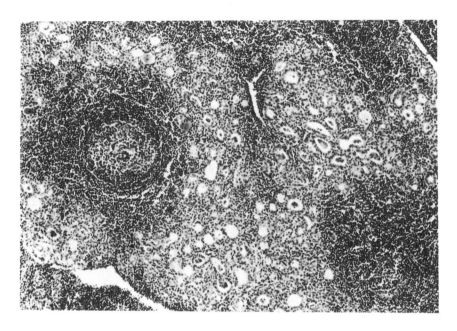

Figure 8.2

432. The likeliest diagnosis is

 (A) granulomatous thyroiditis
 (B) lymphocytic thyroiditis
 (C) nodular goiter
 (D) nodular lymphoma
 (E) Riedel's struma

433. Hypoparathyroidism is most often due to

 (A) accidental removal during thyroid surgery
 (B) autoimmune reaction against chief cells
 (C) developmental failure of parathyroids
 (D) radioactive iodine used in treatment of thyroid carcinoma
 (E) X-radiation to thymus in childhood

The answers are: **426-A; 427-A; 428-E; 429-E; 430-B; 431-E; 432-B; 433-A**. The commonest cause of hyperthyroidism is diffuse hyperplasia (Graves' disease). The hyperplasia is due to the development of autoantibodies to thyroid stimulating hormone (TSH) receptors on the follicular cells. These antibodies cause thyroid hyperplasia and hypersecretion of thyroid hormones. In Graves' disease, the thyroid gland is diffusely and symmetrically enlarged, vascular, and beefy. Microscopically, the amount of colloid is somewhat reduced, and the colloid is scalloped around the edges of the follicles. The cells lining the follicles are enlarged. Papillary projections into the follicles are frequent. Collections of lymphocytes, some having germinal centers, are commonly noted.

Hypothyroidism is a clinical syndrome due to a deficiency of thyroid hormone. It is characterized by a slowing of all body functions. It may occur as a result of congenital absence of the thyroid gland, or it may be due to destructive diseases or total surgical removal of the gland, iodine deficiency, goitrogenic drugs, lymphocytic thyroiditis, or replacement of the thyroid by fibrosis or carcinoma. Radioactive iodine used to treat hyperthyroidism may also cause hypothyroidism.

Myxedema is acquired hypothyroidism. It may occur in children (juvenile myxedema) or in adults. Females are much more frequently affected than males. In fatal cases, the heart may show deposits of mucoid material between the muscle fibers (myxedema heart), pericardial effusion, and cardiac failure. Similar changes occur in the large bowel (myxedema colon). The incidence of atherosclerosis is somewhat increased in patients with hypothyroidism due to the elevated serum cholesterol.

Carcinomas of the thyroid gland, like most thyroid diseases, are more frequent in females than in males. As a class, they are slowly growing neoplasms. Usually they show no endocrine effect. About 60 percent of thyroid carcinomas have a papillary structure, either pure or mixed. Psammoma bodies are frequent in papillary carcinoma. Microscopically, the malignant cells have nuclei with a "ground glass" appearance. Metastasis to the regional lymph nodes is the usual method of spread. The 10-year survival rate is over 85 percent. Previous X-ray therapy to the neck is an important causative factor.

Medullary carcinoma makes up about 5 percent of thyroid cancer and may show an undifferentiated round cell pattern, with stromal amyloid deposits. Electron microscopy indicates that the neoplasm arises from parafollicular C cells. The medullary carcinoma may be a form of carcinoid tumor. It may elaborate an ACTH-like compound, which produces Cushing's syndrome, and calcitonin, as well as serotonin and prostaglandins.

In lymphocytic thyroiditis (Hashimoto's disease), the gland is diffusely enlarged and firm. The acini are almost replaced by great numbers of lymphocytes, often gathered together to form lymph follicles. The surviving acinar epithelium usually is pale and eosinophilic. Lymphocytic thyroiditis is considered to be an auto-immune disorder. Almost all patients have circulating antibodies against thyroglobulin and microsomal antigens of thyroid cells. It occurs in women in over 95 percent of the cases, especially at the menopause.

Hyperparathyroidism may be primary, i.e., due to an adenoma of one or more parathyroid glands, a primary hyperplasia, or rarely a primary carcinoma of the glands; or it may be secondary. The latter is usually associated with chronic renal insufficiency, causing phosphate retention and hypocalcemia with subsequent stimulation of the parathyroid glands. It also occurs with malabsorption and vitamin D deficiency. These glands then become hyperplastic, causing demineralization of bones and elevation of the serum calcium to normal levels.

The pathology of hyperparathyroidism is largely a study of bone changes and of the effects of hypercalcemia. The bones show widespread focal decalcification, followed in some instances by cyst formation, in others, possibly as a result of hemorrhage and minute fractures, by small giant cell tumors composed of osteoclasts, and in still others by fibrosis which obliterates the bony architecture. Reparative giant cell granulomas consisting of fibroblasts, macrophages, osteoclastic giant cells, and blood pigment form brown tumors in bone. The full-blown skeletal disease is called osteitis fibrosa cystica (von Recklinghausen's disease of bone). Hypercalcemia results in deposition of calcium in certain tissues, apparently as a consequence of a local ionic state resulting from the elimination of acid ions. This deposition of calcium in the tissues, metastatic calcification, occurs characteristically in the kidneys, lungs, and stomach.

Hypoparathyroidism is a functional state in which demonstrable organ changes are minimal. The most common cause is accidental removal of the parathyroid glands during neck surgery, particularly thyroidectomy. With hyposecretion of parathyroid hormone there is diminished excretion of phosphorus in the urine, and the serum level rises. The clinical manifestations of hypoparathyroidism are a result of hypocalcemia. When the serum calcium approaches the critical level, increased neuromuscular excitability develops, leading to muscle twitching and occasionally to a convulsive disorder. This excitable state is tetany.

In Items 434-439, match each item with the type or types of diabetes with which it is most closely associated.

        (A)   juvenile onset diabetes mellitus (JOD)
        (B)   mature onset diabetes mellitus (MOD)
        (C)   both
        (D)   neither

434.   hyperglycemia

435.   marked decrease in total islet cell mass

436.   anti-islet cell antibodies

437.   amyloid deposition in islets

438.   insulinitis (lymphocytic infiltration of islets)

439.   gastrin producing islet cell tumor

440.   All of the following are ocular changes in diabetes mellitus **EXCEPT**:

        (A)   cataracts
        (B)   exudates in retina
        (C)   glaucoma
        (D)   microaneurysms in retinal capillaries
        (E)   papilledema

441.   Common findings in cases of diabetes mellitus include all of the following **EXCEPT**:

        (A)   amyloid deposits in glomeruli
        (B)   accelerated atherosclerosis
        (C)   gangrene of the feet
        (D)   hypercholesterolemia
        (E)   increased susceptibility to infections

442. Findings in the offspring of diabetic mothers include all of the following **EXCEPT**:

(A) hyperglycemia
(B) increased incidence of congenital malformations
(C) increased numbers of islets in pancreas
(D) increased risk of hyaline membrane disease of lungs
(E) macrosomia (overweight for gestational age)

ANSWERS AND TUTORIAL ON ITEMS 434-442

The answers are: **434-C; 435-A; 436-A; 437-B; 438-A; 439-D; 440-E; 441-A; 442-A**. In Item 434, hyperglycemia is a feature of both juvenile and mature onset diabetes. In JOD, almost all patients have anti-islet cell antibodies, lymphocytes infiltrate the islets, and there is a marked decrease in islet cell mass. Amyloid deposits are found in hyalinized islets in MOD. Gastrin producing islet cell tumors cause increased HCl secretion by gastric parietal cells and peptic ulcers.

The cause of JOD appears to involve genetic predisposition, virally altered ß-islet cells, and the development of autoantibodies against islet ß-cells. The result is destruction of insulin producing cells. JOD is a much more severe disease than MOD, which usually occurs in older adults. There are genetic factors in MOD, which is mainly due to the development of insulin resistance.

Extensive retinal changes (diabetic retinopathy) occur in diabetics, and may cause blindness. These changes are due, at least in part, to microaneurysms of the retinal capillaries. Hemorrhages, exudates, and microinfarcts also occur in the retina. Organization of a retinal or vitreous hemorrhage may lead to retinitis proliferans, usually 10 to 20 years after the onset of diabetes. Cataracts are frequent in diabetics, due to the conversion of absorbed glucose to sorbitol in the lens, as is glaucoma.

Certain diseases are commonly associated with diabetes mellitus and are generally considered to be complications. Atherosclerosis of medium-sized and large arteries is more common in diabetics than in non-diabetics and occurs at an earlier age. Thrombosis of these vessels is common. Serum lipoprotein and cholesterol levels are often elevated, especially in patients whose diabetes is poorly controlled. Gangrene of the feet in both males and females is commonly of diabetic origin. Capillary basement membrane thickening is found in the skin of the toes of diabetics, as well as in the glomerular and retinal capillaries and elsewhere (diabetic microangiopathy). Diabetics have a general susceptibility to acute infections. In most instances, these infections are due to pyogenic cocci, but there is also a striking increase in fungus infections.

Pregnancy and diabetes present problems to both the mother and the fetus. Acidosis is apt to occur during the last trimester, increasing fetal mortality. Polyhydramnios is very common. The infants of diabetic mothers are often abnormally large. The placenta is increased in size but with immature villi. An increased number of islets of Langerhans is present in the fetal pancreas. Fetal hypoglycemia may develop after birth due to excessive insulin production. Infants born of diabetic mothers are prone to develop hyaline membrane disease. Even with ideal diabetic and obstetric care, fetal mortality is 10 to 15 percent.

CHAPTER IX

NERVOUS SYSTEM PATHOLOGY

Items 443-449

A 20 year-old soldier was brought to the base hospital in a stuporous state. He had awakened that morning complaining of headache and stiff neck. Despite intensive therapy he died the following day. A photograph of his brain at autopsy is shown in Figure 9.1.

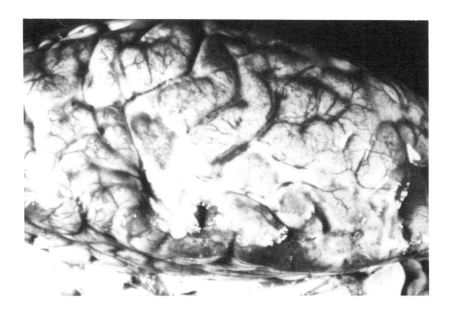

Figure 9.1

443.　The likeliest diagnosis is

    (A)　acute septic meningitis
    (B)　brain abscess
    (C)　fungal meningitis
    (D)　tuberculous meningitis
    (E)　viral meningitis

444. In this case the cerebrospinal fluid (CSF) findings would have shown all of the following **EXCEPT**:

   (A)   1000 WBC/mm^3
   (B)   90% neutrophils
   (C)   glucose 50 mg/dL (normal 40-70)
   (D)   protein 80 mg/dL (normal <40)
   (E)   gram stain - gram-negative diplococci

445. A 20 year-old college student suddenly collapsed. There was a rash. Another student had been hospitalized with meningococcal meningitis. The first student had Waterhouse-Friderichsen syndrome. Its features include all of the following **EXCEPT**:

   (A)   bilateral adrenal hemorrhage
   (B)   infarction of pituitary
   (C)   purpura of skin
   (D)   septicemia
   (E)   shock

446. A 30 year-old man developed headaches and nuchal rigidity. Cerebrospinal fluid examination showed 200 WBC/mm^3, all lymphocytes. The causes of lymphocytic meningitis include all of the following **EXCEPT**:

   (A)   Cryptococcus neoformans
   (B)   Listeria monocytogenes
   (C)   Mycobacterium tuberculosis
   (D)   Treponema pallidum
   (E)   viral meningitis

447. Nervous system lesions which occur in AIDS include all of the following **EXCEPT**:

   (A)   cytomegalovirus encephalitis
   (B)   HIV encephalitis
   (C)   herpes zoster
   (D)   glioblastoma multiforme
   (E)   progressive multifocal leukoencephalopathy (PML)

448. Several years after a case of measles, a 10 year-old girl began to have signs of CNS degeneration. She had most likely developed

    (A)   herpes zoster
    (B)   multiple sclerosis
    (C)   post-infectious encephalomyelitis
    (D)   progressive multifocal leukoencephalopathy
    (E)   subacute sclerosing panencephalitis (SSPE)

449. A 40 year-old man developed convulsions, chills, and fever. A CT scan revealed a spherical lesion in the left cerebral hemisphere. It was diagnosed as a brain abscess. Such a lesion may be secondary to all of the following **EXCEPT**:

    (A)   acute bacterial endocarditis
    (B)   bronchiectasis
    (C)   lung abscess
    (D)   meningococcal meningitis
    (E)   sinusitis

ANSWERS AND TUTORIAL ON ITEMS 443-449

The answers are: **443-A; 444-C; 445-B; 446-B; 447-D; 448-E; 449-D**.

> In Item 443, a soldier living in a barracks who develops headache and neck stiffness is a likely person to have acute septic meningitis, especially meningococcal meningitis. The exact cause would have to be determined by identifying the organism. In acute bacterial meningitis, the CSF glucose level would be markedly decreased.
>
> In Item 445, Waterhouse-Friderichsen syndrome is due to meningococcemia and is characterized by shock and hemorrhages, especially into the adrenal cortices.
>
> Lymphocytic meningitis occurs in tuberculosis, syphilis, fungal infections, and viral meningitides. Listeria causes a neutrophilic response.
>
> Nervous system lesions in AIDS are multifold and due both to the HIV virus itself and opportunistic viral and fungal infections.
>
> SSPE is a slow virus disorder due to measles virus years after the clinical infection or vaccination.
>
> Brain abscess may develop by direct infection during trauma or from the ears or sinuses or hematogenously, most often from lung infections.

Streptococcus pneumoniae, Hemophilus influenzae, and Neisseria meningitidis cause the majority of cases of pyogenic meningitis. Less often the causative organism is another streptococcus, Staphylococcus aureus, Escherichia coli, Pseudomonas aeruginosa, and Listerella monocytogenes.

Meningococcal meningitis is caused by Neisseria meningitidis and is the only type of meningitis having any tendency to be epidemic. Epidemics usually occur in winter, and especially in closed groups such as boarding schools. The organisms apparently enter the bloodstream through the nasopharynx. Bacteremia leads to involvement of the choroid plexus which is followed by meningeal inflammation. The meninges show hyperemia, and a serous to purulent exudate containing PMNs and fibrin collects in the subarachnoid space, especially in the posterior fossa. The blood vessels of the pia-arachnoid are dilated and engorged. The CSF is under increased pressure and is usually cloudy; the cell count ranges from several hundred to thousands of cells/mm^3 (mostly PMNs). Gram-negative diplococci are seen both intracellularly and extracellularly.

In fulminating meningococcemia (Waterhouse-Friderichsen syndrome) there is an abrupt onset of prostration. Cases with adrenal hemorrhages are characterized by shock and an extensive purpuric rash involving the skin and mucous membranes. The hemorrhages are due to disseminated intravascular coagulation triggered by the meningococci.

Besides the lesions listed as occurring in the nervous system in AIDS, toxoplasmosis, many fungus infections, atypical tuberculosis, herpes simplex encephalopathy, lymphomas, Kaposi's sarcoma, and AIDS-dementia complex also have developed.

Slow virus infections of the central nervous system are progressive, degenerative and usually lethal. Progressive multifocal leukoencephalopathy is caused by a papovavirus. This demyelinating disease occurs in patients whose immune response has been impaired by immunosuppression or by a disease such as leukemia or Hodgkin's disease. Intranuclear viral particles are found in oligodendrocytes, the cells which produce and maintain the myelin sheaths. Multiple demyelinated patches are found in the cerebral white matter. The cause of subacute sclerosing panencephalitis (Dawson's encephalitis) has been shown to be measles (rubeola) virus. This disease may occur more than 10 years after the clinical attack of measles. The brain lesions are possibly due to development of an autoimmune reaction. Intranuclear and intracytoplasmic viral particles are found in neurons, astrocytes, and oligodendrocytes. The changes in the brain are similar to those in other types of viral encephalitis plus scattered foci of demyelinization. Kuru and Creutzfeldt-Jakob disease are human subacute spongiform encephalopathies which have been transmitted to experimental animals, although no virus has been identified in brain tissue. Prions have been proposed as the cause. These are proteinaceous infectious particles smaller than viruses. Both diseases are characterized by spongy vacuolation (status spongiosus) of the cerebral and cerebellar gray matter.

A brain abscess is a localized area of suppuration within the substance of the brain. It is usually either cerebral or cerebellar in location. The causative organisms may be introduced by trauma, or by extension from an infection in some adjacent structure, such as the ethmoid or frontal sinuses, mastoid air cells, orbits (abscess), or cavernous sinus (septic thrombosis). In other instances the abscess may be the result of septic embolism during the course of endocarditis, pyemia, or especially pyogenic infections of the thorax (lung abscess, empyema, bronchiectasis, or pericarditis). Streptococci, staphylococci, and Escherichia coli are common infecting organisms. With an abscess the brain is asymmetric in appearance, the affected portion being swollen and the surface markings somewhat obliterated by compression. On section a rounded or ragged cavity is found. It is often lined with a fibrous membrane and filled with creamy pus. Abscesses developing by direct extension are usually solitary; those resulting from septic embolism are often multiple.

192

450. A 40 year-old man suffered loss of deep pain, vibration, and position sense in his legs. Degeneration of the posterior columns in the spinal cord and posterior nerve roots occurs in

    (A) amyotrophic lateral sclerosis
    (B) cerebral infarction involving the internal capsule
    (C) multiple sclerosis
    (D) pernicious anemia
    (E) tabes dorsalis

451. Neuronal loss without inflammation in the anterior horns of the spinal cord is characteristic of

    (A) amyotrophic lateral sclerosis
    (B) cerebral infarction involving the internal capsule
    (C) multiple sclerosis
    (D) myasthenia gravis
    (E) poliomyelitis

452. The development of a tubular cavity in the center of the cervical segment of the spinal cord occurs in

    (A) amyotrophic lateral sclerosis
    (B) acquired immunodeficiency syndrome
    (C) combined degeneration of the cord
    (D) multiple sclerosis
    (E) syringomyelia

453. A 70 year-old woman gradually lost her memory and became unable to care for herself. She was diagnosed as having Alzheimer's disease. Cerebral lesions in this disorder include all of the following **EXCEPT**:

    (A) amyloid deposition in plaques and small blood vessel walls
    (B) areas of demyelinization in gray and white matter
    (C) granulovacuolar degeneration in neurons
    (D) neuritic plaques in gray matter
    (E) neurofibrillary tangles in neurons

454. All of the following are correct statements concerning Huntington's chorea **EXCEPT**:

(A)   it is transmitted as an autosomal dominant
(B)   the disease gene is located on chromosome 4
(C)   the disease becomes manifest in middle life
(D)   neuronal loss is prominent in the caudate nucleus
(E)   the chorea is known as St. Vitus's dance

455. Eosinophilic intracytoplasmic masses (Lewy bodies) in neurons in the substantia nigra are characteristic of

(A)   Alzheimer's disease
(B)   amyotrophic lateral sclerosis
(C)   Huntington's chorea
(D)   multiple sclerosis
(E)   paralysis agitans (Parkinson's disease)

456. All of the following statements concerning multiple sclerosis are true **EXCEPT**:

(A)   grossly gray translucent plaques are scattered asymmetrically
(B)   lesions are more common in white than gray matter
(C)   microscopically demyelinization is a major finding
(D)   plaques are confined to the brain and cranial nerves
(E)   the optic nerves are frequently involved

ANSWERS AND TUTORIAL ON ITEMS 450-456

The answers are: **450-E; 451-A; 452-E; 453-B; 454-E; 455-E; 456-D**.

> Degeneration of posterior columns and posterior nerve roots is characteristic of tabes dorsalis, the spinal form of CNS tertiary syphilis. Quiet degeneration of anterior horn occurs in amyotrophic lateral sclerosis (Lou Gehrig's disease). A tubular cavity in the cervical segment of the spinal cord develops in syringomyelia.
>
> Alzheimer's disease is a dementia characterized by neuronal degeneration in the cerebrum, with amyloid deposition, neurofibrillary tangles, and plaques.
>
> Huntington's chorea is an inherited disease which does not become manifest until adulthood. It is a dementia characterized by neuronal loss.
>
> Parkinsonism in its idiopathic form is typified by neuronal degeneration and pigment loss in the substantia nigra with eosinophilic Lewy bodies in remaining neurons.
>
> Multiple sclerosis is protean in that it involves gray and white matter asymmetrically in the brain and spinal cord. Plaques of demyelinization are typical.

Tabes dorsalis (locomotor ataxia) is neurosyphilis principally involving the spinal cord. It is a late manifestation of syphilis, appearing 10 to 15 years after the primary lesion. It is much more common in males than females. The pia mater is thickened over the affected portions of the spinal cord and may be adherent. The surface of the posterior columns is flattened. The lumbar segments of the spinal cord are mainly involved. The posterior nerve roots are shrunken and gray. There is a degeneration and disappearance of fibers of the lower afferent neurons of the posterior columns. The posterior nerve roots show changes similar to those in the columns.

Amyotrophic lateral sclerosis (ALS) is a chronic, progressive, idiopathic disease with degeneration of the lower and upper motor neurons and marked muscular atrophy. It is more common in males by 4:1 and usually appears in the fourth and fifth decades. A marked loss of anterior horn cells in ALS leads to atrophy of the anterior horns. Many cells disappear, and the remaining ones show all degrees of degeneration. The pyramidal tracts degenerate, and there is a corresponding involvement of the Betz cells of the motor cortex. The motor nuclei of the pons and medulla degenerate late in the course.

In Alzheimer's disease the cerebral cortex is atrophic, especially in the frontal, temporal, and parietal lobes. Senile (neuritic) plaques, found in the cerebral gray cortex, especially in the hippocampus, consist of tangles of unmyelinated axonal processes with a few myelinated axons and rare glial cells. They contain amyloid. Other changes in the cerebral cortex in Alzheimer's disease are granulovacuolar degeneration in the cytoplasm of neurons and the deposition of amyloid in the walls of small blood vessels. Small hemorrhages result from vascular rupture. Increased levels of aluminum have been found in the brains of some patients with Alzheimer's disease. Patients with Down's syndrome show lesions of Alzheimer's disease by age 35. In familial Alzheimer's disease, there is a gene defect on chromosome 21.

Huntington's chorea is a rare hereditary disease transmitted as an autosomal dominant gene. A deficiency of GABA in the corpus striatum and substantia nigra occurs in this disease. Males and females are affected about equally. The disease becomes manifest in middle life. The choreiform movements are probably a result of loss of controlling influences from the neostriatum. Atrophy of some cerebral cortical neurons and degeneration and disappearance of the cells of the putamen and caudate nucleus occur. Death usually occurs in the sixth decade. Huntington's disease gene has been located on chromosome 4.

Parkinson's disease is the result of degenerative changes in the basal ganglia and substantia nigra. Most cases are idiopathic. Tiny golden-yellow lacunae are found in the caudate and lenticular nuclei. There is a loss of dopamine content in the striate body and substantia nigra. Lewy bodies (intracytoplasmic eosinophilic masses with a dark central zone and clearer periphery) are common in the neurons of the substantia nigra. There is neuronal loss and decreased neuromelanin in the substantia nigra.

Multiple sclerosis is an idiopathic, chronic disease of the nervous system characterized by curious remissions and relapses and by the presence of numerous areas of demyelinization scattered throughout the white and gray matter of the brain and spinal cord. The lesions are firm, well-defined, gray, translucent plaques, scattered asymmetrically throughout the central nervous system. They are especially numerous in the pons, medulla, and cerebellar peduncles, and are common in the optic nerve and chiasm. In the spinal cord they are frequent in the lateral columns (pyramidal tracts), and they are not uncommon in the posterior columns. The lesions are found more frequently in the white than in the gray matter of the CNS. There are demyelinization, chronic inflammation, and gliosis. Myelin peels off the axis cylinders, which remain intact for some time.

457. A 35 year-old woman with mitral stenosis and atrial fibrillation suddenly developed left sided paralysis. It was diagnosed as being due to cerebral embolism. Such an embolus most commonly impacts in a branch of the

    (A)   anterior cerebral artery
    (B)   basilar artery
    (C)   lenticulostriate artery
    (D)   middle cerebral artery
    (E)   posterior cerebral artery

458. An 80 year-old man suffered a cerebrovascular accident with left hemiplegia. The cause was a cerebral hemorrhage. Such bleeding frequently originates in the

    (A)   basal ganglia and internal capsule
    (B)   frontal lobe
    (C)   midbrain
    (D)   occipital lobe
    (E)   temporal lobe

459. The causes of cerebrovascular accidents (strokes) include all of the following **EXCEPT**:

    (A)   embolism in a cerebral artery
    (B)   hemorrhage into a glioblastoma multiforme
    (C)   rupture of an atherosclerotic intracerebral artery
    (D)   spontaneous subarachnoid hemorrhage
    (E)   thrombosis of an atherosclerotic cerebral artery

In Items 460-465, match each item with the type or types of bleeding with which it is most closely related.

    (A)   epidural hemorrhage
    (B)   subdural hemorrhage
    (C)   both
    (D)   neither

460. compression of underlying brain

461. grossly bloody cerebrospinal fluid

462. increased intracranial pressure

463. rupture of berry aneurysm of circle of Willis

464. skull fracture

465. venous bleeding

In Items 466-471, match each item with the type or types of injury with which it is most closely related.

        (A)   coup injury to brain
        (B)   contrecoup injury to brain
        (C)   both
        (D)   neither

466. cerebral concussion

467. cerebral contusion

468. epidural hemorrhage

469. fall on back of head

470. impact of blunt object on stationary head

471. subdural hematoma

ANSWERS AND TUTORIAL ON ITEMS 457-471

The answers are: **457-D; 458-A; 459-B; 460-C; 461-D; 462-C; 463-D; 464-A; 465-B; 466-D; 467-C; 468-A; 469-B; 470-A; 471-C.**

Most cerebral emboli enter the middle cerebral artery, apparently because it is the straightest course. The commonest site of cerebral hemorrhage is the basal ganglia and internal capsule due to bleeding from a lenticulostriate artery. These small branches come off the middle cerebral artery under high pressure at a right angle.

Cerebrovascular accidents (CVA's) result from embolism, thrombosis, or hemorrhage. Bleeding into a neoplasm is not a CVA.

Both epidural and subdural bleeding compress the underlying brain and cause increased intracranial pressure. Bleeding does not reach the subarachnoid space, so the CSF is not bloody.

Epidural hemorrhage is due to a sphenoid bone fracture. Subdural hematoma may be associated with a skull fracture but often occurs without one. It is due to venous bleeding.

A blunt object striking the non-moving head causes a coup injury, while a fall on the back of the head results in contrecoup trauma. Epidural hemorrhage is coup, on the side of the causative fracture and arterial tear. Subdural hematoma and cerebral contusion may result from either type of injury. Concussion is not related to either type specifically.

Cerebrovascular accidents include all lesions resulting from damage to blood vessels which produces infarction or hemorrhage in or about the brain or spinal cord. The major types are cerebral infarction and cerebral hemorrhage. Subarachnoid hemorrhage may be spontaneous, especially in patients with hypertension, but is usually due to rupture of or leakage from an aneurysm.

Cerebral infarction results from the occlusion of a cerebral artery due to thrombosis or embolism. Thrombosis, the more common cause, may occur in a cerebral artery damaged by atherosclerosis, periarteritis nodosa, thromboangiitis obliterans, or syphilitic arteritis. Cerebral atherosclerosis is the most frequent cause of thrombosis, common sites of occlusion being the middle cerebral, posterior cerebral, and basilar arteries. Atherosclerosis occurs in the large arteries at the base of the brain.

Embolism in cerebral arteries most often originates from a thrombus in the left side of the heart, in a pulmonary vein, or in other veins by paradoxical embolism. Atheromatous plaques dislodged from the intima of the aorta or a carotid artery by erosion or surgical manipulation may lodge as emboli in cerebral arteries. Embolism is most frequent in branches of the middle cerebral artery, probably because it is a direct continuation of the internal carotid artery. It may produce sudden death without infarction. Multiple small vessel occlusions are common with cerebral embolism. Transient ischemic attacks (TIA's) may result from these.

If the patient survives at least several hours, cerebral infarction often follows cerebral arterial occlusion. The infarct early shows slight softening (encephalomalacia) and a transient infiltration by PMNs. There is degeneration of neurons, axis cylinders, and glial cells, with liquefaction of the lipid material of the myelin. Later, the necrotic material is removed by micro-glial cells which develop a vacuolated cytoplasm (Gitterzellen). Large infarcts have cystic centers filled with yellowish fluid and surrounded by glial tissue.

Cerebral hemorrhage varies from tiny petechiae to massive hematomata. Small hemorrhages result from poisons such as carbon monoxide, bacterial toxins, or purpuric conditions, such as leukemia. Large hemorrhages result from vascular disease, especially atherosclerosis. The most common site of rupture is a lenticulostriate branch of a middle cerebral artery, with hemorrhage into the basal ganglia and internal capsule. In large hemorrhages, the brain bulges on the affected side with flattening of the gyri. The hemorrhage dissects through the brain tissue and may rupture into a ventricle, causing gross blood to appear in the cerebrospinal fluid. A ventricular cast may be formed by clotted blood. Rupture onto the surface of the brain produces subarachnoid hemorrhage. In the hemorrhagic area, there is complete disintegration of brain tissue.

Coup injury is a contusion or laceration of the brain occurring beneath the area of impact on the scalp. It is caused by the impact of a moving object on the stationary head or by striking the head against a sharp object such as a table edge or open drawer. Contrecoup injury is a type of contusion or laceration which occurs opposite the point of impact. Thus, a fall on the back of the head results in contrecoup lesions at the tips of the frontal and temporal lobes where the brain is forced against the irregular bone of the anterior and middle cranial fossae. In such injuries, subdural hematoma, subarachnoid hemorrhage, cerebral contusion, and intracerebral hemorrhage may develop through the coup-contrecoup mechanism. Contrecoup injuries occur exclusively when the head is in motion, at which time the brain tends to lag behind the moving skull. When the skull is abruptly stopped by impact against an immobile object, the lagging brain is struck by the wall of the skull opposite to the area of impact. The pole of the brain diametrically opposed to the point of impact is contused by striking a bony prominence during a gliding motion initiated by the impact. A secondary wave then flows back in the opposite direction toward the impact site, and this may thrust the brain surface there against a bony prominence and produce coup injury.

Cerebral contusion is due to the momentary pressing of the skull against the meninges and brain at the time of impact. It may be coup or contrecoup in type. Multiple contusions of varying ages are common in chronic alcoholics. Early there are characteristic hemorrhages arranged in parallel rows at the peaks of the gyri.

Epidural (extradural) hemorrhage is usually due to fracture, most commonly of the greater wing of the sphenoid bone in the region where the anterior branch of the middle meningeal artery courses through the bone. The hemorrhage is arterial in over 90 percent of cases. A firm clot is usually found overlying the outer dural surface. The underlying brain is indented and hemorrhagic and it may show cortical softening due to venous infarction.

Chronic subdural hematoma results from rupture of a small or large bridging vein crossing the subdural space from the arachnoid membrane to the dura mater. Trauma to the head, sometimes of an apparently trivial nature, is the underlying cause. The cerebrospinal fluid is under increased pressure and is clear or xanthochromic. Following the injury, a clot forms in the subdural space loosely attached to the dura and arachnoid. Within 24 hours, proliferation of fibrous tissue from the dura begins, and in 3 to 4 weeks the clot is covered by fibrous tissue, forming a thin sac filled with dark brown fluid or clotted blood.

A 50 year-old man developed headaches, vomiting, apathy, convulsions, and papilledema. The lesion was determined to be inoperable. He died despite decompression. A photograph of his brain at autopsy is shown in Figure 9.2.

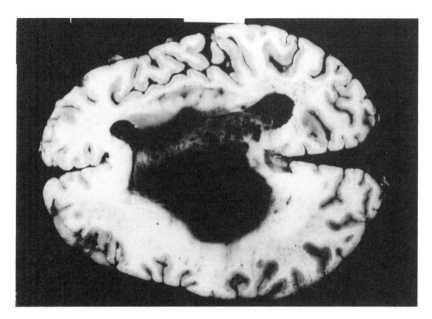

Figure 9.2

472.   The likeliest diagnosis is

    (A)   astrocytoma
    (B)   cerebral hemorrhage
    (C)   glioblastoma multiforme
    (D)   medulloblastoma
    (E)   metastatic carcinoma

473. All of the following statements concerning neoplasms of the central nervous system are true **EXCEPT**:

(A) about half of primary brain tumors arise from glial cells
(B) frequency of CNS tumors is about evenly divided between brain and spinal cord
(C) malignancy of CNS tumors depends on rapidity of growth and location
(D) metastases outside the CNS are rare
(E) the most common source of metastases to the brain is bronchogenic carcinoma

474. A 12 year-old child developed headaches, vomiting, and a staggering gait. A cerebellar neoplasm was diagnosed. The neoplasm which characteristically occurs in the cerebellum in children is

(A) ependymoma
(B) glioblastoma multiforme
(C) medulloblastoma
(D) neuroblastoma
(E) oligodendroglioma

475. A malignant neural neoplasm arising in the adrenal medulla in a child is the

(A) astrocytoma
(B) glioblastoma multiforme
(C) medulloblastoma
(D) neuroblastoma
(E) pheochromocytoma

ANSWERS AND TUTORIAL ON ITEMS 472-475

The answers are: **472-C; 473-B; 474-C; 475-D**.

In Item 472, the clinical signs indicate that a space-occupying mass was present in the brain. The photograph shows a neoplasm involving both cerebral hemispheres and containing a large hemorrhage. These features fit glioblastoma multiforme best.

Neoplasms may occur in the CNS and PNS and their coverings. Most neoplasms of the nervous system are derived from the supporting structures, especially glial cells. Metastasis outside of the central nervous system is extremely rare in primary neoplasms. Spread within the central nervous system is usually via the subarachnoid space, but such spread is commonly localized. Metastases to the brain are common, especially from bronchogenic carcinomas. Medulloblastoma is the commonest cerebellar neoplasm and the neuroblastoma from the adrenal medulla in children.

Glioblastoma multiforme (astrocytoma, grades III and IV) is the most malignant of all brain neoplasms. About 90 percent occur in the cerebrum. The majority of cases occur in the 45 to 55 year age group, and the survival period after diagnosis is usually less than a year. This neoplasm is an irregular, partly hemorrhagic and necrotic, yellow, brown, or reddish gray expansile mass, often measuring up to 5 cm. in diameter. Infiltration across the corpus callosum into the opposite hemisphere is common. The tumor is pleomorphic, with spongioblasts, gemistocytic astrocytes, multinucleated giant cells with bizarre mitotic figures, and a marked increased in vascular elements with endothelial proliferation in the capillary walls.

Medulloblastoma ia a highly malignant neoplasm of children. It originates from residua of the external granular layer of the cerebellum. Medulloblastoma occurs in the posterior vermis and, less often, in the hemispheres of the cerebellum. The medulloblastoma is often circumscribed. It most commonly arises in the midline cerebellum, and usually grows into the fourth ventricle, producing internal hydrocephalus. It is pinkish gray and soft. The typical cell is small and oat- or carrot-shaped with a hyperchromatic nucleus. Clusters of these cells often form pseudorosettes. The medulloblastoma may spread via the cerebrospinal fluid, forming secondary nodules in the brain and spinal cord.

Neuroblastoma is a highly malignant neoplasm which occurs in infants and young children. Its origin is from migrant neuroblast cells in the adrenal medulla, paraganglia, and sympathetic ganglia. In about 40 percent of cases, the neuroblastoma develops in the adrenal medulla. Occasionally a neuroblastoma has matured to a ganglioneuroma through the intermediate stage of a ganglioneuroblastoma. The neuroblastoma is soft, white or yellow, and hemorrhagic; fibrous septa lobulate the mass. The typical cell is small and has a large nucleus and scanty cytoplasm with short processes. Rosette formations are scattered throughout the section.

Metastases to brain are fairly common, occurring in about 20 percent of all fatal malignant neoplasms. About 20 percent of intracranial neoplasms are metastatic. Malignant cells reach the brain by hematogenous routes, especially via cerebral arteries but also through the veins of Batson which drain into the vertebral veins; by direct invasion; and by meningeal spread. The most common source of brain metastases is bronchogenic carcinoma. Other frequent primary sites are the mammary glands, kidneys, skin (melanoma), and gastrointestinal tract. Within the brain, metastatic tumor is usually found in the cerebrum. The metastatic lesions are very often multiple. They are usually well-defined and unencapsulated. Lesions tend to occur at the junction of gray and white matter where blood vessels turn, so that malignant cells may become caught. Edema of cerebral tissue may be striking about metastatic nodules.

CHAPTER X

MUSCULOSKELETAL, CUTANEOUS, AND SENSORY PATHOLOGY

Items 476-485

476.   A 10 year-old boy developed a purulent infection of the skin following an injury. While he was under treatment he began to have pain in the right tibia. An X-ray revealed a focus of bone loss near the upper end of the tibia. Hematogenous osteomyelitis was diagnosed. All of the following are true statements about hematogenous osteomyelitis **EXCEPT**:

   (A)   long bones of the extremities are most often involved
   (B)   bacteria tend to lodge in the metaphysis
   (C)   a fragment of dead bone in the lesion is a sequestrum
   (D)   an increased incidence of osteogenic sarcoma occurs in sites of osteomyelitis
   (E)   Staphylococcus aureus is the commonest causative organism

477.   A fracture in which there are three or more bone fragments is

   (A)   comminuted
   (B)   complete
   (C)   compound
   (D)   pathologic
   (E)   stressed

478.   A 10 year-old boy fractured his right humerus in a fall. The fracture did not heal properly. All of the following are complications of fractures **EXCEPT**:

   (A)   fat embolism
   (B)   hemorrhage between fractured bone ends
   (C)   infection
   (D)   injury to blood vessels and nerves
   (E)   ischemic contracture

479. The most common malignant neoplasm of bone is

   (A)   chondrosarcoma
   (B)   giant cell tumor
   (C)   metastatic carcinoma
   (D)   multiple myeloma
   (E)   osteogenic sarcoma

In Items 480-485, match each item with the type of bone or joint neoplasm to which it is most closely related.

   (A)   chondrosarcoma
   (B)   Ewing's sarcoma
   (C)   giant cell tumor
   (D)   osteogenic sarcoma
   (E)   synovial sarcoma

480.   arises in diaphysis of long bones

481.   arises from osteoclasts

482.   metastasizes to other bones

483.   occurs in increased incidence in osteitis deformans

A 75 year-old woman slipped and fell on her right hip, breaking the femoral neck. She developed pneumonia and died. A segment of her vertebrae is shown in Figure 10.1.

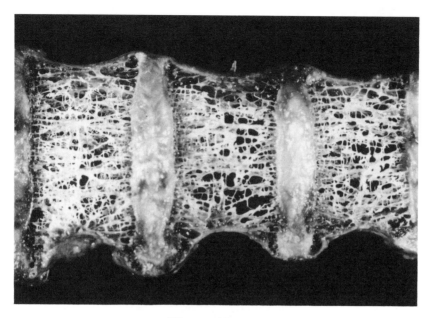

Figure 10.1

484. All of the following statements about the disorder shown in her bones are true **EXCEPT**:

(A)   it is characterized by an absolute loss in bone mass
(B)   it commonly involves the pelvic bones
(C)   fractures and collapse of bone are due to formation of cysts in rarified bone
(D)   it occurs in immobilized bones
(E)   it occurs in Cushing's syndrome

A 20 year-old man developed a swelling above the knee. X-rays showed a mass which had destroyed cortical bone and extended into the surrounding soft tissue. A biopsy revealed marked cellular pleomorphism with numerous multinucleated tumor giant cells. A photograph of the amputated specimen is shown in Figure 10.2.

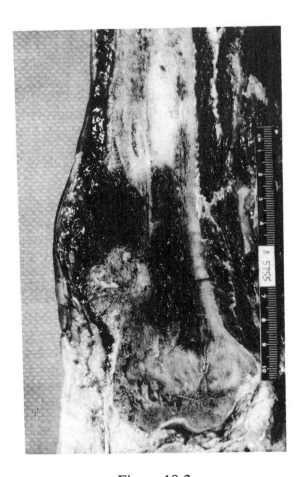

Figure 10.2

485. The likeliest diagnosis is

   (A)   chondrosarcoma
   (B)   endothelial myeloma
   (C)   giant cell tumor
   (D)   metastatic carcinoma
   (E)   osteogenic sarcoma

ANSWERS AND TUTORIAL ON ITEMS 476-485

The answers are: **476-D; 477-A; 478-B; 479-C; 480-B; 481-C; 482-B; 483-D; 484-C; 485-E**. Acute osteomyelitis is a pyogenic infection of bone and bone marrow. It may be a result of direct implantation of bacteria via a puncture wound, extension from an adjacent soft tissue infection, or hematogenous dissemination. While osteomyelitis may occur at any age, the fulminating hematogenous form is more commonly observed in children and adolescents, especially boys. Staphylococcus aureus is the commonest cause.

The long bones of the extremities, especially the tibiae, femora, and humeri, are the ones usually affected in the hematogenous form. Bacteria tend to lodge in the metaphysis. They spread along the small channels within the bone and a purulent exudate forms, burrowing in all directions and elevating the overlying periosteum. Pressure builds up in the tissue spaces as the pus collects. Arteries and veins become compressed and thrombosed, bone cells die and disappear from the lacunae, and eventually the fine osteoid of the bone becomes eroded and liquified.

In fulminant cases the septic thrombi in the venous channels of bone become softened by the action of bacterial and leukocytic enzymes, and embolism to the lungs occurs. The resulting infarcts of the lungs are septic, leading to the formation of multiple abscesses. The usual course is for the infection to spread locally in the bone, causing the death of small bone fragments from ischemia. If the periosteum remains viable, new bone will then be formed, repairing the defect. If the periosteum has been destroyed, or if the necrosis extends up to the articular cartilage, large fragments of dead bone (sequestra) may remain in the area, preventing normal healing of the part and acting as foreign bodies in the wound.

A fracture is designated as simple when the bone is separated into only two parts. When there are three or more bone fragments, the fracture is called comminuted. If the break extends only part way through the bone, it is an incomplete fracture. Types of incomplete breaks include fissure fracture, in which a transverse or longitudinal crack develops partly through a bone; and greenstick fracture, which is caused by marked bending of bone and in which the bone is broken on the convex but not on the concave side. A break produced by slight trauma in a diseased area in a bone, as in a cyst or neoplasm, is called a pathologic fracture. When a piece of broken bone pierces the skin surface, the term compound (open) fracture is applied.

Osteoporosis (shown in Fig. 10.1) is a metabolic disease of bone in which osteoid formation is defective. There is an absolute reduction in bone mass. Osteoporosis is contrasted with rickets and osteomalacia, in which the osteoid is normal but mineralization is deficient. In most cases of osteoporosis, the vertebrae are the bones first and most severely affected, next the pelvic bones, and then the long bones of the extremities. The most common form of osteoporosis is that encountered in older people. This form begins earlier (age 40 to 50) in women than in men and in them is commonly called postmenopausal osteoporosis. Fracture of the femur following a fall is an especially common manifestation. Shortening of stature and limitation of movement due to kyphosis may develop later. Osteoporosis also occurs in Cushing's syndrome, steroid therapy, hyperthyroidism, diabetes mellitus, and immobilized bones.

Metastatic tumors of bone are much more common than primary tumors, especially after middle age. Carcinomas of the prostate often metastasize to the bones of the pelvis and lower spine. Carcinomas of the lungs, breasts, thyroid gland, and kidneys also metastasize to bone.

Giant cell tumor of bone (osteoclastoma) occurs chiefly in young adults, more often in females than males. Its common sites are the epiphyses of long bones, especially at the knee. The giant cell tumor has a soap bubble appearance on X-ray. Normal bone is replaced by soft, yellowish red granular tissue. Hemorrhages in the tumor are common, but fractures are rare. The distinctive cell is the osteoclastic giant cell. About 30 percent recur after removal, and about 20 percent metastasize.

Of the malignant tumors primary in bone, the most important is the osteogenic sarcoma. It has one peak of incidence in the second and third decades, and another in later life, the latter apparently being secondary to chronic bone disease, particularly Paget's disease of bone and radiation osteitis. Important sites of occurrence of osteogenic sarcoma are the ends of the long bones (85%), particularly about the knees. In some cases, there is a soft bloody lesion destroying bone (osteolytic) and invading the soft tissues, whereas in other cases the periosteum is elevated as a result of the formation of sclerotic new bone. Microscopically, the pattern is also extremely variable both from case to case and also from area to area in the same case. This pleomorphism is one of the most distinctive microscopic features of the neoplasm. Multinucleated tumor giant cells are numerous. Spindle-shaped connective tissue cells are also common. In the more sclerotic types, imperfect new bone trabeculae may be recognizable. Venous invasion occurs early, often leading to widespread pulmonary metastases.

Chondrosarcoma is a malignant neoplasm arising in bone, occurring usually about age 45. It is three times as common in men as in women. Its usual site is at the end of a long bone. It is a lobulated tumor which often extends along the marrow cavity for some distance, eroding bone cortex and bulging into the soft tissues. Microscopically, the resemblance to the cells and matrix of hyaline cartilage is usually clear, even in those cases in which calcification and ossification have occurred.

Ewing's sarcoma is a rare neoplasm, occurring in males more often than in females and chiefly at age 10 to 25. It often occurs on the diaphyses of long bones. It is a soft gray tumor which arises in marrow, erodes the bone cortex from within, and often causes new bone formation beneath the periosteum. It is composed of uniform small cells resembling lymphocytes. Metastases often appear in other bones, a feature rarely noted in other neoplasms primary in bone, and in the lungs. Its histogenesis is uncertain although recent evidence suggests a neuroectodermal derivation.

Items 486-496

486. All of the following occur in Reiter's syndrome **EXCEPT**:

   (A)   conjunctivitis
   (B)   gonorrhea
   (C)   HLA-B27 histocompatibility type
   (D)   polyarthritis
   (E)   urethritis

In Items 487-492, match each item with the type or types of arthritis with which it is most closely related.

   (A)   osteoarthritis
   (B)   rheumatoid arthritis
   (C)   both
   (D)   neither

487. damage to joint cartilage

488. Heberden's nodes

489. bacterial infection of synovia

490. IgM antibodies against altered IgG

491. sequela of rheumatic fever

492. synovial pannus formation

493. All of the following statements are true concerning ankylosing spondylitis **EXCEPT**:

   (A)   it is especially common in persons of HLA-B27 histocompatibility type
   (B)   it leads to ankylosis of intervertebral joints
   (C)   it occurs much more frequently in men than in women
   (D)   it may cause restricted pulmonary ventilation
   (E)   it is associated with an increased incidence of osteitis deformans

494. A 50 year-old man suffered from classic primary gout, especially after voluminous eating and drinking. All of the following statements about this disorder are true **EXCEPT**:

(A) it almost always occurs in men
(B) it is inherited as an X-linked disorder
(C) the metatarsophalangeal joint of the great toe is classically involved
(D) tophi made up of urate crystals and foreign body giant cells are common
(E) tophi often occur in the ears

495. Atrophy of muscle fibers due to lower motor neuron loss occurs in

(A) amyotrophic lateral sclerosis
(B) Guillain-Barré syndrome
(C) myasthenia gravis
(D) syringomyelia
(E) tabes dorsalis

496. All of the following statements about Duchenne muscular dystrophy are true **EXCEPT**:

(A) it is transmitted as an X-linked recessive
(B) onset is at 3 to 6 years of age
(C) muscle involvement is asymmetrical
(D) the pelvifemoral muscles are involved early
(E) pseudohypertrophy of the calf muscles is common

ANSWERS AND TUTORIAL ON ITEMS 486-496

The answers are: **486-B; 487-C; 488-A; 489-D; 490-B; 491-D; 492-B; 493-E; 494-B; 495-A; 496-C**. Reiter's syndrome (RS) is characterized by polyarthritis, non-gonococcal urethritis, and conjunctivitis. About 70 percent of patients have the HLA-B27 antigen. The cause of urethritis is most often Chlamydia trachomatis or Ureoplasma urealyticum. In RS, knees, ankles, feet, and wrists are involved asymmetrically. The arthritis is aseptic and may be caused by immune complex deposition. The synovium is infiltrated by neutrophils. There is little or no synovial cell hyperplasia until late, when lymphocytic infiltration occurs.

Rheumatoid arthritis is a chronic inflammatory disease of the joints. It affects women chiefly and has its onset characteristically in middle life. Its cause is most likely an autoimmune reaction. The changes in the joints vary with the stage of the disease. Punch biopsies of the synovium show varying degrees of proliferation of synovial cells and fibroblasts, disarrangement of collagen fibers, edema, increased vascularity, and minimal cell infiltration, consisting chiefly of lymphocytes and plasma cells. The former are mainly T lymphocytes. In more advanced cases, the synovium forms a thickened pannus, and the articular cartilage becomes eroded to bone. Subcutaneous rheumatoid nodules occur in 25 percent of the cases. The center of the nodule is generally necrotic, eosinophilic, and somewhat granular (fibrinoid necrosis). This area is surrounded by a zone of radially arranged elongated cells resembling the epithelioid cells of a tubercle, with lymphocytes and plasma cells interspersed. Nodules also occur in the myocardium, aorta, and lung. The heart shows endocardial or pericardial lesions in some cases. Rheumatoid factor is present in about 75 percent of cases. It is an IgM antibody against IgG produced by plasma cells in synovia.

Degenerative joint disease (osteoarthritis) is the most common of all types of joint disease. Some degree of joint degeneration is inevitable with aging. Due to the friction of weight bearing and motion and to the loss of elasticity in the cartilage, there is thinning of the articular cartilage, leading to narrowing of the joint space and to loss of stability. These changes in turn lead to erosion of the cartilage. Cartilage does not regenerate following injury. Bone, as it becomes exposed on the joint surface, reacts to form bony spurs (osteophytes). This leads to irregularity of the joint surfaces and to further fragmentation, so that particles of bone and cartilage break loose into the cavity (joint mice). The polishing of exposed and thickened bone by wear is eburnation.

Ankylosing spondylitis is characterized by inflammation of the cartilaginous joints between the vertebral bodies and of the gliding joints between the vertebral arches of the spine. It leads to progressive fibrous ankylosis of the cartilaginous joints, often with kyphosis so severe that patients cannot raise their heads. Kyphosis also leads to restriction of rib mobility and impaired pulmonary ventilation. This in turn may lead to cor pulmonale and heart failure. Men are affected about 8 times as often as women. About 90 percent of patients have the HLA-B27 histocompatibility type.

Classic primary gout is a constitutional disorder occurring in males in about 95 percent of the cases. It is manifest by joint disease and is associated with an inherited defect of purine nucleotide metabolism which is transmitted polygenically. The disease occurs in two forms: acute gouty arthritis, in which there is sudden severe inflammation, usually of a single joint, and chronic tophaceous gout, in which there are multiple joint deformities and extensive deposits of urates in the tissues.

The acute attack often follows a period of excessive eating or drinking. It often begins abruptly at night, as acute inflammation of the metatarsophalangeal joint of one of the great toes. Serum uric acid levels are markedly elevated during the acute attacks. After 10 years or so, about half the patients who have recurrent attacks of gouty arthritis develop chronic tophaceous gout. The urate deposits occur in the hands and feet, and the skin over the large nodular lesions sometimes ulcerates. The deposits in the synovial membranes and articular cartilages cause a progressive deforming arthritis. Gout seems to predispose its victims to vascular disease. Hypertension commonly occurs, and often causes death from coronary or cerebral thrombosis in the sixth or seventh decade.

The lesions of chronic tophaceous gout are firm nodular masses (tophi) beneath the skin of the ears, in the periarticular tissues of the fingers, toes, and elbows, and in the synovial membranes and articular cartilages of the large joints. Sheaves of urate crystals can be demonstrated in tissues. Polarized light reveals doubly refractile crystals. Foreign-body giant cells, lymphocytes, and macrophages occur at the periphery of the tophi. Similar, although smaller, deposits of urates are frequently noted in the renal medulla. In about 10 percent of fatal cases, uric acid calculi will be found in the urinary tract.

Atrophy is the muscle change resulting from interruption of the motor nerve supply, whether in the motor cortex, the lateral columns, the anterior horn cells of the spinal cord, or the peripheral nerves. The diseases of the nervous system are primary and the muscular weakness is secondary. Atrophic fibers are scattered among normal fibers. In amyotrophic lateral sclerosis or poliomyelitis, an entire mass of muscle fibers may show atrophy, and may eventually almost disappear.

Much more complex is the genetically determined condition known as progressive muscular dystrophy. A number of different forms have been described, affecting different muscle groups and having onset at different ages. The pseudohypertrophic form of Duchenne is the most common. It symmetrically affects chiefly the pelvifemoral muscles, with onset at about 3 to 6 years and death before age 20. Inheritance of the Duchenne type is by an X-linked recessive. Microscopically, in muscular dystrophy there is a broad range of changes in muscle, from almost no abnormality in the youngest individuals affected to almost complete replacement of muscle bundles by adipose and fibrous tissue in the older patients. The essential change is degeneration of the muscle fibers. In the pseudohypertrophic type, extremely large muscle fibers are mingled with narrow atrophic fibers.

In Items 497-504, match each item with the dermatitis or dermatosis with which it is most closely related.

        (A)   acne vulgaris
        (B)   acute dermatitis due to poison ivy
        (C)   dermatitis herpetiformis
        (D)   erythema multiforme
        (E)   lichen planus
        (F)   pemphigus vulgaris
        (G)   pityriasis rosea
        (H)   psoriasis
        (I)   seborrheic keratosis
        (J)   urticaria pigmentosa

497.   delayed hypersensitivity reaction

498.   dense dermal infiltration by mast cells

499.   herald patch

500.   IgA deposits along basal layer of epidermis

501.   large bullae on skin and oral mucosa

502.   papules and pustules on skin of face

503.   sprue-like pattern in jejunum

504.   violaceous papules on forearms and wrists

505.   All of the following are associated with an increased incidence of epidermoid carcinoma of the skin **EXCEPT**:

        (A)   acne vulgaris
        (B)   arsenic
        (C)   ionizing radiation
        (D)   methoxypsoralen therapy
        (E)   ultraviolet radiation

506. All of the following are correct statements concerning malignant melanoma of the skin **EXCEPT**:

(A)   ultraviolet sunlight is an important causative factor
(B)   light-skinned individuals have a higher incidence that dark-skinned ones
(C)   it arises from melanocytes in the basal layer
(D)   it spreads via lymphatics early, then hematogenously
(E)   it occurs in increased incidence in patients with AIDS

507. All of the following are characteristic of basal cell carcinoma **EXCEPT**:

(A)   deep invasion
(B)   lymph node metastases
(C)   multicentricity
(D)   occurrence on skin of face
(E)   ulceration

ANSWERS AND TUTORIAL ON ITEMS 497-507

The answers are: **497-B; 498-J; 499-G; 500-C; 501-F; 502-A; 503-C; 504-E; 505-A; 506-E; 507-B**. Psoriasis is a common chronic, recurrent skin disease which is sometimes associated with arthritis. It may be a disorder of epidermal cell replication. The number of basal cells is increased, and the time of cell passage from basal layer to stratum corneum is only 3 days (normal 27 days). The extensor surfaces of the elbows and knees are most commonly affected, but the entire skin may be involved. The lesions tend to be symmetrical and grossly are sharply outlined, dry, red to brown papules and plaques covered with fine silvery scales.

Acute dermatitis occurs in the contact reaction due to poison ivy and to other agents. It is a delayed hypersensitivity reaction. There is intense itching and even burning. The affected skin areas are swollen, reddened, and vesiculated. The vesicles are intra-epidermal, with cellular necrosis. The superficial dermis has edema, capillary dilatation, and perivascular infiltration with neutrophils, eosinophils, and lymphocytes.

Dermatitis herpetiformis is chronic, recurrent, and characterized by itching. It is often associated with persons with HLA-B8. Deposits of IgA are found along the basal layer in skin adjacent to the lesions. There is a symmetrical distribution of groups of papules, vesicles, and, rarely, bullae surrounded by zones of erythema. These lesions occur most commonly on the shoulders, extensor surfaces of the extremities, and the buttocks. Microscopically, the epidermis is only slightly affected, but there is subepidermal vesicle formation with a marked neutrophilic and eosinophilic infiltrate of these lesions and the surrounding dermis. Some patients with dermatitis herpetiformis have a sprue-like pattern in the jejunum, and DH appears to be due to a gluten hypersensitivity.

Pemphigus vulgaris is a severe bullous dermatitis characterized by itching and burning. It occurs most often in the fifth through the seventh decade of like. The skin of the axilla and groin is particularly affected, however, any part of the skin may be involved. Oral lesions often appear first. The bullae are soft and break easily, releasing fluid with an offensive odor. Degenerated squamous cells (Tzanck cells) are found singly and in clusters within bullae. In pemphigus vulgaris IgG autoantibodies against an antigen in intercellular spaces and circulating autoantibodies are found.

Erythema multiforme is an acute dermatosis which is part of a self-limited systemic disease with fever and sore throat. It is most commonly idiopathic, but may be drug-induced or following herpes simplex. The skin lesions are pleomorphic with macules, papules (the commonest manifestations), vesicles, and bullae. The papules often enlarge peripherally and clear centrally to form the typical iris lesions. The vesicles and bullae form by complete separation of the epidermis from the dermis.

Acne vulgaris is a persistently chronic disorder which usually appears during adolescence, involving the face and upper chest and back. Sebaceous gland ducts become blocked, and sebum accumulates. When sebaceous follicles rupture, keratin in the comedos stimulates foreign body reactions. Lipolytic enzymes elaborated by bacteria act on lipids in sebum to release free fatty acids, which mediate papule and pustule (pimple) formation. The papules show a lymphocytic and plasmacytic infiltrate, with occasional foreign body giant cells about pilosebaceous glands which contain inspissated sebum. Bacterial infection, often by <u>Corynebacterium</u> <u>acnes</u> or <u>Staphylococcus</u> <u>epidermidis</u>, causes pustulation and subcutaneous abscesses. In the later stages, dermal fibrous scarring develops in some of the lesions.

Pityriasis rosea is probably due to a virus and usually lasts 4 to 6 weeks. The disease occurs most often in the spring and summer in children and young adults. It begins with a patch on the trunk, followed by the appearance of numerous round, pinkish buff patches on the trunk. Thin scales overlie the lesions. There are occasional small vesicles in the epidermis.

Lichen planus is idiopathic, persists for months or years, and usually causes severe pruritus. The flexor surfaces of the wrists, forearms and legs often have small, angulated, plateau-like violaceous papules. A heavy lymphocytic infiltrate is present in the upper dermis and crowds up against the epidermis.

Epidermoid carcinoma of the skin constitutes about 15 percent of all cancer in males and 10 percent in females and causes about 2 percent of cancer deaths. Certain factors are related causally: ultraviolet rays; chronic irritation; ionizing radiation; carcinogenic hydrocarbons; and arsenic. An increase in squamous carcinoma occurs in patients treated for psoriasis with high doses of methoxsalen (methoxypsoralen) and UV photochemotherapy.

Epidermoid carcinoma occurs most commonly on the exposed surfaces (such as the face or hands), especially over bony prominences. Early there is slight thickening of the skin or mucosa. Later an ulcer with thick, indurated edges appears and will not heal. Columns, sheets and clusters of atypical squamous cells invade the dermis. Metastases are mainly to regional lymph nodes, but late in the course metastases may be widespread.

Basal cell carcinoma metastasizes extremely infrequently. It occurs predominantly in fair-skinned persons on the region of the face bounded by the hairline, ears, and upper lip. Its origin is from the cells of the basal layer of the epidermis or the hair follicles. Basal cell carcinoma is a slowly growing lesion, beginning as a papule which soon ulcerates centrally. The ulcer border is waxy and rolled. The neoplasm, if neglected, may eventually erode deeply and invade the underlying bone. The lesions may be multiple. Solid sheets of small, hyperchromatic, basophilic cells extend in columns from the epidermis into the dermis. The columns often have club-shaped endings.

Malignant melanoma arises from melanocytes in the skin or uveal tract, and rarely from the conjunctiva and other mucous membranes. The highest incidence is in fair-skinned people. Excessive exposure to ultraviolet rays in sunlight is a predisposing factor.

Three forms of melanoma occur. Lentigo maligna melanoma arises in a melanotic freckle of Hutchinson in elderly persons. It is usually on a cheek or other exposed surface and invades only after months or years. Superficial spreading melanoma, the commonest type, grows laterally and invades late. Nodular melanoma invades early and shows no adjacent intra-epidermal component. It has a worse prognosis than the other two forms.

Melanoma is either elevated (nodular) or flat (lentigo maligna and superficial spreading), and is usually darkly pigmented. Signs of malignancy in a pigmented skin lesion include variegated color, an irregular border, and an uneven surface. In invasive melanoma, sheets and clusters of atypical polyhedral or spindle cells arise from the lower epidermal layers and invade the dermis. The cells are commonly loaded with melanin. Some melanomas are excised before dermal invasion has occurred or extended beyond the papillary dermis (superficial melanoma). In these cases, there is marked junctional activity with many atypical melanocytes containing melanin granules in an otherwise clear cytoplasm. In the underlying dermis in melanoma, there is marked infiltration of lymphocytes and plasmacytes, and numerous pigment-laden macrophages are seen.

Spread is via lymphatics early, with later extensive hematogenous dissemination. Regional lymph nodes are involved frequently. Hematogenous metastases are common in the skin, lungs, liver, intestines, heart, adrenals, kidneys, and brain.

Items 508-517

508.   The causes of granulomatous inflammation of the inner eye include all of the following **EXCEPT**:

(A)   gonococcal ophthalmitis
(B)   histoplasmosis
(C)   sarcoidosis
(D)   sympathetic ophthalmitis
(E)   toxoplasmosis

509.   All of the following statements about sympathetic ophthalmitis are true **EXCEPT**:

(A)   association with an anterior perforating wound in one eye
(B)   bilateral uveal granulomas
(C)   immune reaction to uveal pigment protein develops
(D)   prompt enucleation of wounded eye is preventative
(E)   there is an increased incidence of ocular melanoma

216

510. The causes of glaucoma include all of the following **EXCEPT**:

   (A)   abnormally narrow anterior chamber angle
   (B)   defective formation of the anterior chamber angle
   (C)   particulate matter in trabecular meshwork
   (D)   retinal detachment
   (E)   synechiae in an anterior chamber angle

511. The causes of lenticular cataract include all of the following **EXCEPT**:

   (A)   diabetes mellitus
   (B)   intraocular foreign body containing iron
   (C)   maternal rubella in first trimester of pregnancy
   (D)   oxygen therapy in a premature infant
   (E)   senile degeneration

512. A middle-aged man suddenly lost a field of vision. Ophthalmoscopic examination revealed a retinal detachment. The causes of such a detachment include all of the following **EXCEPT**:

   (A)   contraction of a vitreous fibrous band
   (B)   fluid accumulation behind the retina from a choroidal melanoma
   (C)   fluid accumulation behind the retina from hypertensive retinopathy
   (D)   decreased intraocular pressure (hypotony)
   (E)   retinal hole or tear

513. A premature infant was treated with increased oxygen concentrations because of respiratory distress. A few months later it was noted that the child was blind. The ocular lesion induced by oxygen therapy is

   (A)   congenital cataracts
   (B)   congenital glaucoma
   (C)   granulomatous endophthalmitis
   (D)   interstitial keratitis
   (E)   retrolental fibroplasia

514. A 2 year-old child became blind in the right eye and showed a yellow "cat's eye" reflex when light was shone into the pupil. Ophthalmoscopic examination revealed a white mass projecting from the retina. Retinoblastoma was diagnosed. All of the following are true statements about retinoblastoma **EXCEPT**:

   (A)   about half of cases are inherited as an autosomal dominant
   (B)   some cases have a deletion in the long arm of chromosome 13
   (C)   it arises from retinal neuroblasts
   (D)   malignant cells are often arranged in rosettes
   (E)   it is highly malignant and metastasizes widely

515. Of the following, the one statement which is true concerning ocular melanoma is

   (A)   it is more common among African-Americans than whites
   (B)   it may arise from the iris, ciliary body, or choroid
   (C)   extension is common along the optic nerve
   (D)   rosette formation is a characteristic microscopic finding
   (E)   foci of necrosis and calcification are common in the tumor

516. Papilledema of the optic nerve head is caused by

   (A)   increased intracranial pressure
   (B)   increased intraocular pressure
   (C)   physiologic variation
   (D)   systemic hypertension
   (E)   trauma

517. A 28 year-old composer began to lose his hearing first in one ear then bilaterally. By his 40's he was almost totally deaf. Otosclerosis has been considered a likely cause. All of the following statements about otosclerosis are true **EXCEPT**:

   (A)   it is inherited as an autosomal dominant
   (B)   bony lesions resemble osteitis deformans
   (C)   hearing loss is due to ankylosis of the stapes in the fenestra ovale
   (D)   attacks of vertigo with nausea and vomiting are common
   (E)   tinnitus occurs in most patients

ANSWERS AND TUTORIAL ON ITEMS 508-517

The answers are: **508-A; 509-E; 510-D; 511-D; 512-D; 513-E; 514-E; 515-B; 516-A; 517-D.**
Granulomatous endophthalmitis occurs in tuberculosis, leprosy, sarcoidosis, syphilis, brucellosis, fungus infections, toxoplasmosis, helminthic infestations, sympathetic ophthalmia, and phacoanaphylaxis (a complication of cataract). In the infectious forms, the organisms usually reach the inner eye hematogenously. Hypersensitivity plays a role in causing tissue damage in many forms of uveitis.

Sympathetic ophthalmitis (sympathetic uveitis) is the development of a bilateral granulomatous inflammation of the uveal tract following a perforating wound of the anterior segment of one eye. If the wounded (exciting) eye is not promptly enucleated, sympathetic uveitis follows about 5 percent of such injuries, and blindness may result in the opposite (sympathizing) eye. The lesion apparently is an auto-immune reaction to released uveal pigment protein. Microscopically, the uveal tissues are densely infiltrated by lymphocytes with islands of epithelioid cells. Eosinophils are occasionally numerous.

Glaucoma is a complex of diseases characterized by an elevated intraocular pressure. The normal range is 12 to 20 mm. of mercury. Glaucoma is usually caused by a decrease in the outflow of aqueous humor.

Congenital glaucoma is usually transmitted as a simple recessive trait. Boys are affected about twice as often as girls. Some cases are due to maternal rubella. The condition is bilateral in about 65 percent of cases. The cornea becomes hazy and cloudy due to edema. The most consistent finding is an anterior insertion of the iris on the trabecular meshwork. Late in the course of congenital glaucoma the eye becomes very large in all directions (buphthalmos) since all coats stretch readily in infancy.

Primary closed-angle glaucoma is paroxysmal, occurs in women more often than in men, and is related to the development of an abnormally narrow anterior chamber angle. The attacks are usually unilateral at first, but later occur bilaterally. The anterior chamber loses depth with age, due to enlargement of the lens. Highly hyperopic eyes are especially prone to acute angle closure glaucoma due to an associated narrow angle. In acute glaucoma, the eye is stony hard and markedly congested with dilated pupil and edematous cornea. In mid-dilation of the pupil, the iris may contact the forwardly placed lens, causing a partial pupillary block. As posterior chamber pressure rises the peripheral iris is bowed forward. Then there is contact between the iris and trabecular meshwork. Early there are no actual adhesions, but with long contact peripheral anterior synechiae develop. The meshwork undergoes fibrosis and degenerative changes, and Schlemm's canal is compressed and later obliterated.

Primary open-angle glaucoma (chronic simple glaucoma) is a progressive disease in which the anterior chamber angle may vary from excessively wide to somewhat narrow. The disease is bilateral and increases in severity and frequency with age. This form makes up over 60 percent of glaucoma in adults. It is significantly associated with myopia, diabetes mellitus, and the inability to taste phenylthiocarbamide. Most cases of chronic simple glaucoma are probably inherited as a recessive trait. Clinical signs and symptoms usually do not appear before 40. The principal pathologic changes are probably in the trabecular meshwork due to degeneration and sclerosis of its collagen fibers, especially those adjacent to Schlemm's canal.

The intertrabecular spaces adjacent to the canal are narrowed and even closed. However, these changes could be an effect rather than the cause of the increased pressure.

Secondary glaucoma is usually unilateral. It is almost always due to changes in the anterior chamber. Secondary angle-closure glaucoma may result from pupillary block in iritis and partial lens dislocation, or following cataract extraction (due to forward protrusion of the vitreous face). Angle closure is most often due to the formation of peripheral anterior synechiae, as in acute and chronic iridocyclitis; penetrating wounds; contusion; vascular disease of the posterior segment of the eye; and intraocular neoplasm (by pushing the iris forward, an associated iridocyclitis, or invasion of the angle).

Secondary open-angle glaucoma is due to particulate matter in the trabecular meshwork. In acute iridocyclitis, inflammatory cells may block the meshwork, but glaucoma is not common because aqueous production is decreased. Glaucoma is more common in chronic anterior uveitis. Trauma is an important cause; glaucoma may result from erythrocytes in the meshwork or clotted blood in the angle resulting from anterior chamber hemorrhage in ocular contusion. Penetrating injuries may lead to epithelial or endothelial proliferation over the meshwork, although peripheral anterior synechia formation and angle closure is a more common cause following such injuries.

The effects of glaucoma on ocular tissues are widespread and may be severe. The corneal epithelium becomes edematous in acute or chronic glaucoma. Lens cataract is often present in long-standing glaucoma. The iris shows ischemic necrosis in acute glaucoma due to interference with its nerve and blood supply. The entire uveal tract becomes atrophic in long-standing glaucoma, the choroid being least affected. The retina shows degenerative changes in the nerve fiber and ganglion cell layers with gliosis. The optic disk is cupped.

A cataract is an opacity of the lens often due to the accumulation of interfibrillar fluid and the precipitation of proteins within the lens. Cataract may be congenital or it may be due to trauma; intraocular inflammation; physical agents such as ionizing and microwave radiation, infrared radiation and electric shock; intraocular foreign bodies containing toxic metals (iron, copper); drugs such as adrenocorticosteroids; diabetes mellitus; tetany; and, most commonly of all, senile degeneration.

Senescent cataract occurs because of degenerative changes in persons beyond middle age. Two forms occur; the nuclear (sclerotic) and the cortical (liquefactive). In nuclear sclerosis, there is gradual enlargement, increased yellowness and density, and loss of transparency of the nucleus. Occasionally the nucleus or even the entire lens becomes dark brown or black. In the cortical type, fluid accumulates in and between lenticular fibers early. With time the fibers become edematous and fragmented.

The complications of cataract are phacogenic glaucoma and endophthalmitis. Glaucoma may be due to interference with intraocular fluid flow by pupillary block due to a markedly swollen cataract, or by escaped liquefied lens protein from hypermature cataracts. This fluid is phagocytized by macrophages which plug the anterior chamber angle (phacolytic glaucoma). Phacoanaphylactic endophthalmitis is due to a hypersensitivity reaction to released lens protein. A tuberculoid granulomatous reaction occurs on the surface of the lens and around separated lenticular fragments in the vitreous or aqueous humor. Synechiae plaster the lens to the iris.

Detachment of the retina is a separation of the neuroepithelial layers from the pigment epithelium layer, thus depriving the former of an adequate blood supply. Such a detachment is due to the accumulation of fluid in the potential space between these two portions of the retina, a vestige of the central cavity of the embryonic optic vesicle. Fluid accumulations may come about by extravasation from the choroid or retina in chorioretinitis, choroidal or retinal neoplasms, hypertensive retinopathy, or retinal venous occlusion; by the contraction of vitreous fibrous bands which have been formed following intraocular trauma, inflammation, neovascularization, or hemorrhage and are attached to the inner retina, the contraction pulling apart the layers of the retina; or by the pouring of fluid from the vitreous into the space through a retinal hole or tear (rhegmatogenous retinal detachment). Such retinal openings may occur following ocular contusion or mild trauma, especially in myopic eyes, or they may develop spontaneously. Once vitreous fluid seeps through a retinal defect, it spreads through the subretinal space, peeling off more of the neural retina.

Retrolental fibroplasia is an oxygen-induced degeneration in the premature infant in whom the peripheral retina is not completely vascularized. In such an infant, an increased oxygen tension causes immediate but transient closing down of terminal arterioles and the arterial side of the capillary bed. With continued increased oxygen levels an irreversible vaso-obliteration occurs. The involved vessels degenerate, and vasoproliferation from adjacent vessels begins. Newly formed capillaries invade the retina, penetrate the internal limiting membrane, and grow into the vitreous. Retinal detachment may be caused by organization of vitreous hemorrhages and exudates and the formation of a preretinal membrane. In severe cases, a completely detached retina and organized vitreous form an opaque retrolental mass giving a white cat's-eye reflex (leukocoria).

Retinoblastoma is the most common malignant intraocular neoplasm of infancy and childhood. It arises from retinal neuroblasts and probably has it inception during intrauterine life, although it is usually not apparent at birth. Retinoblastoma occurs with equal frequency in boys and girls. In some cases, there is a deletion from the long arm of chromosome 13 (13q14). About 40 percent of retinoblastomas are inherited as an autosomal dominant with strong penetrance, and half of such cases are bilateral. In about 20 percent of all cases of retinoblastoma, the neoplasm is bilateral. The mortality rate is about 10 percent, most deaths occurring within a year after discovery. The pupil of the involved eye becomes white or gray, and a yellow reflex is seen behind the pupil when light is shone into it (amaurotic cat's-eye reflex). Ophthalmic examination reveals a white or gray mass projecting from the retina.

Retinoblastoma usually arises in the posterior retinal hemisphere. It may grow mainly endophytically into the vitreous humor with seeding onto the lens, ciliary body, and iris or exophytically with invasion of the subretinal space and choroid. In either form, secondary foci of tumor tissue are common on the retina and the optic disk. Extension is common along the optic nerve. Microscopically, the retinoblastoma consists of small cells with prominent, hyperchromatic nuclei. In well-differentiated examples, there are numerous Flexner-Wintersteiner rosettes in which the cells are arranged circularly with their cytoplasmic processes extending centrally. Foci of necrosis with calcification are common in retinoblastomas.

Ocular melanoma may arise from the iris, ciliary body, or choroid. It is rare in African-Americans. Choroidal melanoma early is a disk-shaped, pinkish to dark brown mass located most commonly in the posterior segment. Eventually it breaks through the lamina vitrea and invades the retina, forming a mushroom-shaped mass. Uveal melanoma shows plump spindle-shaped cells with a large, prominently nucleolated nucleus. Necrosis is not common.

Extraocular extension of melanoma may occur in cases of choroidal melanoma. The periorbital tissues may be invaded through the sclera or by means of emissary veins. Distant metastases are hematogenous and are most common in the liver.

Papilledema is a swelling of the optic nerve head usually produced by stasis in the central retinal vein caused by increased intracranial pressure. Another factor is the transmission of the elevated intracranial pressure along the meningeal sheaths of the optic nerves. Occasionally sudden hypotony resulting from intraocular surgery or from a penetrating eye wound results in papilledema. As fluid collects, the nerve fibers become edematous. The retina is pushed away from the disk margin by the fluid accumulation and becomes folded.

Otosclerosis is an osteodystrophy of the bony capsule of the inner ear that may produce progressive bilateral deafness. The cause is uncertain, but otosclerosis appears to be inherited as an autosomal dominant trait with limited penetrance. The disease is as common in women as in men. The bony lesions resemble those of osteitis deformans. There is lacunar absorption of the bone of the otic capsule with replacement by immature, vascular spongy new bone. This is resorbed and replaced by more mature, web-like, lamellar bone. These gradual resorptions and replacements produce a mosaic pattern. Later the involved bone becomes dense, avascular, and eosinophilic, the sclerotic phase of the disease. The process usually begins in the bone between the fenestra ovale and cochlea. Deafness begins when the process involves the foot plate of the stapes in the fenestra ovale and produces bony stapes ankylosis which interferes with the transmission of sound waves to the perilymph of the cochlea.